POSITIONING YOUR PRACTICE FOR THE
MANAGED CARE MARKET

Glenda

For your library

Tom

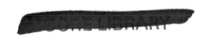

POSITIONING YOUR PRACTICE FOR THE MANAGED CARE MARKET

EDITED BY

J. Thomas Danzi, M.D., F.A.C.P.
Vice President and Medical Director
Senior Associate Dean for Clinical Affairs
Hahnemann University Hospital
Medical College of Pennsylvania/Hahnemann
University School of Medicine
Philadelphia, Pennsylvania

Editor: David C. Retford
Managing Editor: Kathleen Courtney Millet
Production Coordinator: Kimberly S. Nawrozki and Linda Carlson
Copy Editor: Anne K. Schwartz
Designer: Norman W. Och
Illustration Planner: Raymond Lowman
Typesetter: Peirce Graphic Services, Inc.
Printer: Victor Graphics

**W
130
AA1
P8
1996**

© Copyright 1996 Williams & Wilkins

351 West Camden Street
Baltimore, Maryland 21201-2435 USA

Rose Tree Corporation Center
1400 North Providence Road
Building II, Suite 5025
Media, Pennsylvania 19063-2043 USA

Accurate indications, adverse reactions, and dosage schedules for drugs are provided in this book, but it is possible that they may change. The reader is urged to review the package information data of the manufacturers of the medications mentioned.

Printed in the United States of America

Library of Congress Cataloging-in-Publication Data

Positioning your practice for the managed care market / edited by J. Thomas Danzi.
    p.   cm.
    Includes index.
    ISBN 0-683-02373-X
    1. Managed care plans (Medical care)—United States. 2. Medicine—Practice—United States. I. Danzi, J. Thomas.
    [DNLM: 1. Managed Care Programs—United States. 2. Practice Management, Medical—trends—United States. W 130 AA1 P8 1996]
    RA413.5.U5P67 1996
    610'.68—dc20
    DNLM/DLC
    for Library of Congress   95-44935
                                                    CIP

                                            96 97 98 99 00
                                 1 2 3 4 5 6 7 8 9 10

Reprints of chapter(s) may be purchased from Williams & Wilkins in quantities of 100 or more. Call Isabella Wise, Special Sales Department, (800)358-3583.

PREFACE

Managed care has had a great impact on the practice of medicine and medical practice. The medical profession has lost its autonomy and fiscal control of the delivery of health care in this country. Physicians are being unilaterally excluded from participating in managed care health plans with no due process proceedings.

Evidence suggests an excess of specialists in this country by the end of this century. Specialists are retraining to primary care physicians. The unthinkable of a nonreimbursed practicing physician has become a reality.

The intent of *Positioning Your Practice for the Managed Care Market* is to educate physicians about managed care, managed care contracts, and the evaluation of their care provided by managed care companies. It is hoped that the readers will be in the best position to ensure their participation and success in the new health care marketplace.

J. Thomas Danzi, M.D.

ACKNOWLEDGMENTS

I wish to express my gratitude to my wife, Betty, for her understanding and encouragement in the completion of this literary project. I wish to also thank our children, Carolyn, Kori, and Jay, for their support and understanding of the time commitment necessary to complete this book.

I would like to acknowledge the coordinating and transcriptional support provided by Anita Delquadro, which allowed this literary project to be efficiently completed.

CONTRIBUTORS

Thompson H. Boyd III, M.D.
Attending Physician, Hahnemann University Hospital
Department of Medicine
Hahnemann University Hospital
Philadelphia, Pennsylvania

Joseph R. Carver, M.D.
Medical Director, U.S. Healthcare
Blue Bell, Pennsylvania
Associate Professor of Clinical Medicine
Cardiovascular Institute
Hahnemann University
Philadelphia, Pennsylvania

Peter Chodoff, M.D., M.P.H.
Professor of Anesthesia
Jefferson Medical College
Special Projects, Health Policies and Clinical Outcomes
Thomas Jefferson University Hospital
Philadelphia, Pennsylvania

J. Thomas Danzi, M.D., F.A.C.P.
Vice President and Medical Director
Senior Associate Dean for Clinical Affairs
Hahnemann University Hospital
Philadelphia, Pennsylvania

Carolyn L. Danzi, M.D.
First Year Resident
Department of Pediatrics
Georgetown University Medical Center
Washington, DC

Alice G. Gosfield, J.D.
Alice G. Gosfield and Associates
Past President, National Health Lawyers Association, 1992–1993
Member, Board of Directors, National Committee for Quality Assurance
Philadelphia, Pennsylvania

Harry Gottlieb, M.D.
Senior Vice President and Senior Associate Dean for Clinical Affairs
Professor of Medicine
Medical College of Pennsylvania Hospital
Philadelphia, Pennsylvania

Judy B. Harrington, M.B.A.
Senior Vice President, Managed Care
Allegheny Integrated Health Group
Allegheny Health, Education and Research Foundation
Adjunct Faculty
Health Administration
Temple University
Philadelphia, Pennsylvania

Christopher G. Lang, J.D.
Warner and Stockpole
Boston, Massachusetts

Jonathan L. Lord, M.D.
Executive Vice President
Anne Arundel Health Care System
Annapolis, Maryland

David Nash, M.D., M.B.A.
Associate Professor of Medicine
Jefferson Medical College
Director of Health Policies and Clinical Outcomes
Thomas Jefferson University Hospital
Philadelphia, Pennsylvania

Christopher E. Nolin, J.D.
Warner and Stockpole
Boston, Massachusetts

Neil Schlackman, M.D., F.A.A.P.
President, USQA
Medical Director, US Healthcare
Blue Bell, Pennsylvania

CONTENTS

IV / Legal Implications of Managed Care
115

V / Perspectives of Managed Care
185

□

SECTION ONE

THE REALITY OF MANAGED CARE

□

CHAPTER ONE

INTRODUCTION

J. Thomas Danzi

The 1992 presidential campaign and President Clinton's promise to enact health care reform forced many physicians to realize that the golden era of fee-for-service medical care was soon to be over. The reality of a managed care–dominant health care market seemed destined to be the national standard. When Congress was unable to enact health care legislation in 1994, some physicians mistakenly assumed that the issues of access to health care, the prohibitive cost of health care delivery, and the increasing penetration of managed care in the health care marketplace would somehow be resolved with no impact on them. The truth is that economic and societal factors had already allowed enhanced penetration of the managed care delivery model in many large health care markets in the country. Health care reform is occurring and is being driven by competitive market forces. Any legislated health care reform will address the apparent disproportion of specialists to primary care physicians, ensure access to care for all Americans, and enact cost-control measures.

Many challenges are posed by these changes. How can a primary care or specialist physician understand what managed care companies are seeking in their contractual relationships? Do most physicians know their fixed costs for providing care and the procedures performed? What information is available to address the quality and the clinical outcomes of care provided? Do physicians understand a capitated payment system and risk sharing? What physician-integrated organization is worth joining in a managed care–predominant health care market? These are a few of the important questions that most physicians in this country seek to have answered.

The vast majority of physicians complete their residency training without didactic courses in either medical school or residency training on the economic realities and administrative requirements of clinical practice.

There is a need for curriculum change with the inclusion of health care policy issues, the credentialing process for hospitals and managed care companies, physician participation in quality improvement and utilization review activities, and office management functions. Therefore, it is not surprising that so many physicians are perplexed by the challenges ahead.

In response to these needs, state and national medical societies are developing educational programs for their members. Topics of these seminars include definitions of managed care, understanding health care capitation and risk contracting, practice profitability analysis, office management topics such as time and personnel management, and integrated physician organizations, to highlight a few. I have personally found that personal participation in more than one seminar is usually required for a good working understanding of these important topics. The obvious downside to this approach is the cost associated with lost office revenue and meeting attendance.

In the past decade, an increasing percentage of physicians have entered employment relationships with group practices or health maintenance organizations after completing their postgraduate educational training programs. The three main reasons cited are the provision of a billing/certification function by the institution, the presence of a managed care contract office, and the security of a regular salary. The lack of financial knowledge about managing a practice in this new health care marketplace is making the solo practitioner a possible feature of the past.

Solo practitioners and small group practices are developing different types of physician-integrated organizations to help secure some of the benefits that large group practices offer their physicians. These physician-integrated organizations include independent practice associations (IPAs), preferred provider organizations (PPOs), physician hospital organizations (PHOs), and integrated delivery systems (IDSs). There are advantages and disadvantages to each type of organization, with the latter organizations requiring physicians to leave the autonomy of solo practice and become partners in an organization, with their financial benefits and risks dependent upon the success of the organization.

While attempting to resolve these issues, it is not uncommon to have the hospitals where these practitioners admit patients become involved in different forms of agreement to protect their market niche. The agreements range from generally cooperative to affiliation, merger, or consolidation. The reason for the "mergermania" is usually to reduce administrative overhead, improve negotiating positions with health care payers, or gain access to new health care markets. This compounds the practitioner's insecurity.

Obviously, physicians are seeking answers to many important questions so they can correctly position themselves for financial security in a most complex health care marketplace. This book is intended to enable those practitioners to successfully address many of the perplexing realities they face in medicine today.

□

CHAPTER TWO

REALITY OF HEALTH CARE REFORM

Jonathan L. Lord

The certainty of sustained, accelerating change in society forms the basis of this chapter. It takes little effort to assess history to understand that this has been our heritage. It is more difficult to approach the prospect of change optimistically—although there too, history in the larger sense and our individual personal histories show that we have a remarkable ability to adapt and succeed! The past 100 years have provided examples of the cycle—invention, transition, mass deployment, refinement, invention—for products and services in virtually every aspect of our lives. The primary subject of this book, health services and hospitals, has been through this cycle at least once, and in some aspects (diagnosis and treatment of disease) several times. The hospital as we visualize it today is an invention of this century; our efforts at refinement and invention are our focus.

CORE CHANGES AFFECTING HEALTH CARE TODAY

The issues facing health care can be divided into two major categories:

- Constants of change
- Unique, contemporary pressures

The constants of change relate to those functions that affect all aspects of society. These include the core economic pressure of increasing worker productivity, the constant of technology change and improvement, and an expectation of lifestyle enhancement from generation to generation. It is the unique and contemporary pressures on health care that we need to tease out and use in planning our strategies for the future. These include the following.

The Transition of Focus from "Supply"-Side Services to "Demand" Side.   This transition has been spurred on by a greater sense of the individual's ownership in his or her decision making, a thirst for information and subsequent ability to rapidly access such information, and an ongoing erosion of tolerance of paternalistic behaviors on the part of any "institution" (government, medicine, or corporation). For our field it means leaving the "father knows best" approach behind; it means living the first step of the Alcoholics Anonymous 12-step model by admitting "that we have no control" and orienting our approach to appreciate the role of the "customer" of our services, collaborating with them to design services that meet their needs as opposed to providing those services on the sole basis of our professionally developed model. The potential for inventing great community-focused, community-responsive services in partnership with our neighbors exists only when we recognize the power of this transition.

Moving from "Illness" to "Wellness."   We have "refined" the invention of the hospital around the management of sick people. Our efforts have been based on a premise that health is defined as the absence of illness, and we have done a lot to treat, conquer, and eradicate illness. In other fields we have learned that definitions built on the negative have only limited value. Most of the readers of this book have lived through this in the transformation in the quality field—20 years ago we generally defined quality as the absence of disquality (defects) in contrast to our contemporary understanding of quality improvement theory's multiple dimensions of quality. For many health care professionals, the definition of "wellness" is soft, ambiguous, and "faddish." Later in the chapter we will discuss the definition of health.

Shifting from Discrete Payments for Services for Individuals to Prepaid, Population-based Payment Systems.   This results in a radical rethinking of our business efforts. For years we have focused on the addition of services intended to add revenue (radiology, laboratory, and other procedures) as opposed to efforts to manage the appropriateness and effectiveness of the services provided. We were able to hypertrophy our ability to measure the financial impact of these services without investing in analyzing their impact—as long as we made revenue targets, we were satisfied.

Making Quality a Strategic Imperative.   This is absolutely linked to the movement to demand-side thinking; the notion of providing data about the value of services is critical in today's health care marketplace. For too long, the quality efforts in health care have been delegated by leadership to a group of individuals focused on regulatory compliance and meeting the needs of "alien life forms" that visit health care organizations from time to time (the Joint Commission on Accreditation of Healthcare Organizations, the Healthcare Finance Administration, and state inspec-

tors) instead of designing and building services that exceed the expectations of patients and other customers in the system. Quality measurement
efforts need to focus on value; for the purpose of this chapter, value will
be defined as the relationship of functional and clinical outcomes and patient and other customer perception of services to the cost of services.

The fundamental impact of these highly interrelated core changes is
manifested in the ways we approach our efforts today:

- Contemplating overcapacity and the impact of the shift of risk
- Emphasizing health
- Relationships among practitioners (primary care and specialists)
- Developing data sets to demonstrate value
- Developing networks and collaborating with groups outside of tra-
  ditional health care

DEFINING OUR HEALTH SYSTEM

Discussion of change is not possible without taking an inventory of our
current system for the delivery of health. Again, we must define what we
mean. A close colleague, Gene Beyt, M.D., of Baton Rouge, took the unusual step of asking his patients what they thought health was. The way
he did it was even more unusual—he gave his patients disposable cam-
eras and asked them to take pictures of "health." Much to his surprise,
there were no pictures of hospitals or doctors or nurses. Instead, there
were pictures of kids playing in playgrounds, families going to church together, people exercising, parks, and trees. We have repeated this approach in other communities with similar results. What it allows us to do
is move off the negative definition (health is the absence of illness) to begin to look at health from multiple dimensions (medical, emotional, spir-
itual, financial) that we can positively influence. From this perspective,
our position as the "300-pound gorilla" in the system is dwarfed. We can
begin to recognize that we neither have the "franchise" on health in our
communities (and as a consequence the total accountability for health) nor
the resources ourselves to "fix" health problems. Going back to our 12-
step model, our position should be to influence the direction of our community's health as opposed to "controlling" it.

Something even more remarkable occurs if we step back and look at
how we (hospitals, health systems, and doctors) fit into the health decision-making processes of people. Another colleague, David Sobel, M.D.,
from the Kaiser System, has analyzed people's behaviors and concluded
that more than 80% of health care decisions are self-managed by individuals. A simple way to test this theory with any group that you may be as-

sociated with—church, PTA, group practice—is to ask if they have had a headache, backache, muscle cramp, or stomach ache in the past 2 weeks and follow up by asking how many of those people went to a doctor or emergency room with that complaint. The results are amazingly consistent—very few people accessed the health system to treat their symptoms; instead, they treated themselves and went to the supermarket, the pharmacy, or the health food store to remedy the problem. David estimates that just a 5% increase in self-management could result in nearly a 50% decrease in the consumption of resources from the organized components of the delivery system. Beyond the self-managed component of the health system, there is a "hidden" system of care provided by families and other informal networks. It turns out that if you have some relationship to the organized health system (like being an employee in a hospital or clinic), you can become an "oracle" of health advice to your neighbors. Thus, even a housekeeper in a hospital becomes an important tool in efforts to improve the health of the community.

Other groups involved in health care that "we" (those of us in the organized health systems) don't normally recognize are regularly used by our patients. These include a whole host of "alternate" providers such as those in chiropractic, herbal medicine, diet and nutritional service, massage, and music therapy. A recent *New England Journal of Medicine* article points out that in 1993, nearly 13 billion dollars were spent in this category of services (about 50% of the dollars spent on primary care medical services in the same year!), and nearly 10 billion dollars came out of the pockets of individuals rather than from insurers or the government. We arrive at "us" at the end of the discussion, not because we are the least important, but because we need to begin to understand that we are not the "alpha and omega" of the health care universe but only one (very expensive) part of it. The implication is clear as we approach our strategies for the future:

Strategy development must contemplate integrating or coordinating each one of these aspects (self-management, informal networks, alternate providers, and the visible system) if we are to succeed in improving the health of communities or populations within communities.

STRATEGIES FOR CHANGE

Refinement of today's hospital and health systems requires "drilling down" in five key areas:

- Infrastructure
- Information systems

- Designing care
- Work redesign
- Clinical resources management

The common thread of these efforts is to focus on the core processes or services of the health system and to position the patient and other customers of the system at the point of central focus. As you will see, these efforts are not mutually exclusive but instead build upon one another.

Infrastructure

Infrastructure changes run the gamut from a preeminent focus on quality, to restructuring the core delivery models (such as the critical care, intermediate care, medical-surgical care paradigm), to rethinking reward and recognition programs, to committee and meeting models. An entire book can be written on this subject alone. We will focus on some baseline philosophy, the "how do we start?" issues, and a smorgasbord of examples.

Some basic ingredients are required to make the types of changes that are necessary to be successful in the future. They include a real commitment to the core reason that the enterprise exists (taking care of patients), the engagement and education of the organization's leadership, and memorializing the values of the organization on the basis of values brought by the professional caregivers who make up the majority of the staff. Essential to this effort is an explicit acknowledgment of the need to ask people what they want instead of telling them what they want. With this core in place, it becomes possible to begin to ask the community, key stakeholders, other customers, staff, and organizational leadership: what makes this place essential to us? how does the system impact on our lives? how should it? what would happen if it were suddenly gone? and how would we cope? Asking those questions again and again, allows development of priorities and strategies to accomplish those strategies. While that process is going on, a simultaneous tack is to start examining institutional "stupidities"—the things that every organization has and does without any apparent reason other than "that's the way we have always done it." Easy targets here include committees and their associated meetings—we truly have achieved some unique successes in health care, and one of them is to measure productivity by the number of committees per adjusted occupied bed. Using that measure, we have been fantastic performers, spurred on by the total quality management (TQM) movement, which encouraged work groups, teams, and other "new committees" in addition to our existing efforts. This may be a little "tongue in cheek," but we manage to layer this "stuff" to the point that our decision-making processes look akin to a "cow eating breakfast" (chewing, swallowing, regurgitating, chewing, and the cycle goes on!). Part of the reason to attack this waste is that we really need the time for other things, we need to send some signals of fundamental change and to practice the *power of asking*. In this case we are asking ourselves and others: what can we really eliminate without adversely affecting patient care? With these basics in place, one can work on a variety of infrastructure issues. For example:

- Leadership development and education for the board, medical staff leaders, and management team. Inevitably these efforts lead to systematic personal mastery programs, reassessment of committee and bylaws structures, and evolutionary expansion of physician leadership of organization-wide activities.
- Development of recognition programs that are focused on desired behaviors rather than programs exclusively aimed at identifying and punishing the undesirable behaviors (e.g., programs to reward and recognize the timely completion of medical records vs. focusing on those who do not do so).
- Asking patients and ourselves such questions as "why do we transfer patients in the hospital?" We can ask whether we built a system around the patient or developed a system in which the patient has to conform to our requirements. Among the innovations to come out of these discussions are strategies to decentralize functions or approaches such as "universal" or fungible beds, where the patient is cared for in one location and the technology and staff are rotated around the patient.
- Innovation in programs aimed at creating healthier employees including health risk assessment, incentives for healthier behaviors, and education in self-management of medical and health-related activities.
- Apply management talent to core processes and "outsource" the management of processes outside of clinical care to others (food services, logistics, security, etc.)

Information Systems

Let's begin by saying three times: "information systems, information systems, information systems." There simply isn't any future without effective information systems for two basic reasons:

- We must be able to articulate the value of service. To do that we must have data and we must manage it.
- We must take labor costs out of the system (and thereby drive productivity up).

This doesn't necessarily mean expensive systems, nor does it mean deferring on every issue "until we get a computer." It does mean diagraming core business processes (e.g., how do we manage a patient with gallbladder disease?), identifying where information technologies would facilitate the management of care, and knowing what technologies are available. It also means organizing the collection of data at the most direct, accurate, and timely base ("handle the data/source once"). This will generally tie data collection directly to care provision. Lastly, it means arraying the data and their analysis to be responsive to the demands of the marketplace and usable at all levels within the organization. To those ends, Gene Nelson and Edward McEachern of Dartmouth have developed the concept of a "value compass" that visually depicts the relationship of functional and clinical outcomes, customer (patient) satisfaction, and cost for individual services or service lines. For example, the following types of technology applications and approaches to data management are not grossly expensive yet follow the core processes of what happens in hospitals and health systems.

- *Simulation technologies* allow visualization of how processes perform over time. This type of technology is geared to measuring movements (e.g., of patients, blood specimens, x-rays) through an area of a hospital or clinic (emergency room, operating room, medicine clinic) in relationship to physical layout and staff. Once diagramed, these systems allow diagnosis of inefficiencies and playing "what if" games to test facility or staff redesign.
- *Group systems technologies* are designed to facilitate decision-making processes and to decrease the time spent in meetings. These professionally developed tools have the paradoxical ability to increase participation of staff while decreasing the labor content lost to meetings. They can be used within existing hospital or health system networks or as "stand-alone" systems
- *Comparative databases* come in all shapes and sizes. The obvious benefit is providing external benchmarks of performance. Keys for evaluation include ease of supplying/accessing data, applicability of data displays, richness of database (number of participants and longevity of database), and ability to provide customized comparative reports. The databases tend to be specialized around resource consumption, clinical outcome, or patient satisfaction.
- *Concurrent data collection* means reorienting most of the coding, abstracting, and quality functions of hospitals and clinics to the real time in which the patient is being cared for. The advantages of this process include
  —Decreased rework and handling of records

—Improved accuracy of records through dialogue among clinicians and staff involved in data collection

—Enhancement of case mix

—Timely availability of data

—Faster turnaround times for record completion

- *Voice technologies* will become more prominent and hold hope for order entry, integration into enterprise-wide systems for follow-up (such as automated results from laboratory equipment directly into a physician's voice mail box) and someday soon, automated transcription services.

These are just a few of the systems and approaches that relate directly to the enterprise-wide "legacy" systems that are the basic engine for health systems. Focusing on utility, simplicity, and "real world" applications is the key to the sane deployment of information systems. Linking back to our central theme, *the power is in asking* the right question; in this case, it is how can we make your job better (easier) or how can we make your experience better.

Designing Care

Designing care is a curious phrase. It is my premise that the care delivery system has never been designed; if it was, it was done by a madman. From virtually every perspective—financing, care delivery, and facility—the system is not a system at all, but instead a collection of processes that have been spot welded, wired together, or sometimes just cling to one another. Often we encounter processes that are at complete odds with one another; other times we scratch our heads and ask "why are we doing this." Every health care practitioner can readily identify stupid, redundant, or wasteful practices, yet somehow we do the same thing over and over again. We can't really begin to design care until we have worked on infrastructure and introduced some changes to our technologies. The relationships among these activities are not simple cause and effect, but are more circular, with each step affecting the others. We need to work on infrastructure first because

We need the insight on the part of leadership to trust the notion of *asking* rather than telling.

We need to free up staff's time from wasted meetings to serve on new teams or groups.

The prework that is involved in information systems is related to "cleaning up" the accuracy and timeliness issues in the system, being sure that the information system isn't seen by the practitioners as the "enemy," and having some plan in place for meeting future requirements. Perhaps the most important prework is making sure that organizational leaders are committed to long-term and ongoing investment in technologies as a core cost of doing business in the future.

The process of designing care begins with understanding community and organizational priorities—what are the most important services that the organization provides now or will provide in the future? The process of design is expensive (not necessarily without substantive return) and requires time to accomplish. Efforts need to be related to the priority areas (which are also among the higher-volume areas) of service. Outlining the process is straightforward; accomplishing it is artwork.

- Identify priority areas
- Assemble a group of key stakeholders
- Describe the purpose of the group
- Discuss existing activities
- Dream about future states and diagram how the future state should function
- Simultaneously diagram existing systems, gather literature and performance benchmarks
- Analyze the gap between "ideal" and existing systems
- Prioritize areas for change
- Redesign the system
- Test the redesign with customers
- Refine design on the basis of customer input
- Measure the performance of the new system design
- Continue quality improvement efforts

The "artwork" side of this process cannot be turned into a cookbook. It is related to the leaders' ability to work with and understand people. Hints about things that work that are listed below, but there is no chronological or priority order to them.

- Focus on care (not on finances, not on implementing a program or bureaucratic terminology)
- Include direct caregivers
- Include patients and other customers
- Do not send issues into "bureaucratic black holes" for management approval; have the authority to make resource-based decisions within the team
- Practice looking at things from the converse or challenging current activities with "what if" questions

In previous writings we have described the process of designing care across the continuum of care, with emphasis on the pre-, in, and post-hospital phases of care. For patients with chronic disease, the component of services is particularly important, because they provide the opportunity to keep the patient from decompensating and requiring additional hospitalizations. Examples of design work in our experience have resulted in

- *Measurement of functional outcomes* using modified Harris Hip Scales to assess the improvement in mobility and decrease in pain in total joint replacement patients
- *Development of a cardiac "clinic"* to manage acute chest pain patients and to rule out myocardial infarctions within 18 hours of presentation to the emergency department
- *Admission of patients* directly to their beds from physician offices
- *Redesign of documentation systems* to documentation of exceptions rather than all entries
- *Incorporation of patient satisfaction* measures in the patient's computer-based record
- *Development of universal beds,* eliminating the need to transfer patients

The list goes on and on; not the creation of expensive consultants, but the work of staff who take care of patients every day.

Work Redesign

As we progress through infrastructure change, deployment of information systems, and the design of care, we inevitably get to a point at which we have to confront the way we and our staff work. Once we move from redesign systems that may be remote to the individual and bring change down to an "eyeball-to-eyeball" level, we enter a phase of resistance, fear, and hostility. Generally, as long as change affects someone else, we are champions for change; when change affects us, we argue for the status quo, question our future, and are frightened by ambiguity. This is compounded by a misimpression that we have become conditioned to believe in: that the world moves from one steady state through a period of change to another steady state. Unfortunately for our defense mechanisms, the paradox is that the one constant is change, and the rate of change is constantly accelerating. When we take a step back we can see this in every aspect of our lives, but we don't necessarily know how to harness the energy of this process and instead try to resist it!

Let us inventory the types of work redesign we can see across health care:

- *Physicians* see their work change in a number of dimensions. The development and rapid deployment of new technologies cause physicians to use new medications, to stop doing procedures that they were tried for, and to replace them with new types of procedures (e.g., laparoscopic, minimally invasive procedures) that they have to learn in the middle of their careers. Changes in payment mechanisms cause primary care physicians to manage patients differently, to operate their offices with different types of staff, and to change relationships with specialist physicians. New information technologies that allow patients to complete their own histories, to work through algorithms to determine the need for care, and to interact with their practitioners, without ever coming to the office, radically changes what physicians do in their offices.
- *Nurses and other hospital staff* are radically rethinking their jobs. The development of "patient-focused" and "Planetree" approaches to care tends to consolidate job categories, including some nursing functions, respiratory care, physical therapy, laboratory, x-ray, and to make the contact with patients more intimate. In some institutions, nurses and other staff have begun to use computer devices that are worn on their belts to record vital signs and other patient data, eliminating the need for paper records. First in obstetrics and subsequently in adult medicine, the redesign of facilities to eliminate the need to regularly transfer patients (e.g., labor and delivery to postpartum and newborn units) causes major change in the skill sets and competencies of primary caregivers.
- *Support staff* from physician offices to the hospital are seeing major change. Of particular interest is the measurement of performance, in which traditional job categories in the quality area (quality improvement, risk management, infection control, utilization management) together with coding, abstracting, education, and training are integrated to focus on the design and measurement of performance in clinical areas of the hospital. In such systems, application of the tools of quality improvement and communication of results and strategies for improvement are clinical service functions, not centralized bureaucratic quality functions.

It takes little imagination to understand the tremendous recasting of work that will take place in the near term; it takes a tremendous effort to prepare staff for this much change.

Clinical Resources Management

Clinical resources management is the culmination of these efforts. The concept is based on the principle of "designing in" the use of resources rather than tracking how resources are consumed. These efforts are predicated on team design of care and simplification of measurement systems to focus on points that are important to the ultimate consumer of service (patients and/or beneficiaries) and are responsive to the marketplace. For example, building in the timely and appropriate laboratory workup for preoperative patients so it happens with a key stroke rather than requiring remembering, documenting, validating, and then doing, which necessitates subsequent rechecking to see if the process was done correctly.

FACTORS FOR SUCCESS

There are three points of focus for success in the future. First, focus on patient care (including wellness services), since it is the core process of our field. Second, be true to the values of caregivers—advocate for the needs of people. Third, position the organization to demonstrate the value of its services (functional outcome, clinical outcome, satisfaction, and cost). In attempting to lead organizations through change leaders must

- Focus on health
- Understand and know core processes
- Believe that everyone in the enterprise really wants to do what is right
- Use scientific methods to design and measure services
- Apply the principles of continuous improvement theory

The Chinese character for chaos is also the character for opportunity. Collectively, we can harness the energy of change to create better systems for health and health care.

□

CHAPTER THREE

DEFINITIONS OF MANAGED CARE

J. Thomas Danzi and Judy B. Harrington

As the discussion of health care reform continued, the American public and health care providers had many proposals to consider as the solution to a health care delivery system that had been characterized by high cost, inconsistent outcomes, and poor preventive health programs. The proposals varied from a form of socialized medicine with a single-payer government-based health delivery system to a market-driven managed health care delivery system or the managed-competition approach, which relies on a combination of market forces and government regulation. The challenge was to thoroughly understand each proposal: what it meant, what the governmental role was, what changes should result, and how it would affect the purchasers, patients, and providers of health care.

Not infrequently, the public and providers heard or read about recommendations made by the Jackson Hole Group, the Pepper Commission, the Advisory Council on Social Security, and the National Leadership Coalition for Health Care Reform. There were comparisons with the socialized health care systems of Canada, Japan, Germany, and Great Britain. There were at least 14 health care bills introduced in Congress since 1991. The public and providers were trying to understand the "alphabet soup" of provider groups, including HMOs, PPOs, IPAs, and MSOs. Finally, a new glossary of health care terms evolved, which included *capitation, bundled payments, discounted fees, risk sharing, open and closed HMOs, lock-ins, deductibles and authorization review,* to name a few. We were pleased, yet amazed, that Congress decided it was best not to enact some type of health care reform at the end of the 1994 session. The American public, health care providers, and members of Congress needed more time to make an educated decision about which reform bill should be passed or whether it was best to let market forces change the health care delivery system.

This chapter presents an overview of managed care, an understanding of the differences between managed care and managed competition, a glossary of key managed care terms, and the stages of penetration of managed care in the marketplace, highlighting the significance of each stage for physicians.

A broad definition of *managed* care is health care that focuses on high-quality cost-efficient care with emphasis on the preventive and wellness aspect of health. The care is commonly delivered by a health maintenance organization (HMO), which is a legal entity that provides or arranges for the provision of covered health services to a defined population for a predetermined fixed prepaid premium. This definition of an HMO was taken from the HMO Act of 1973 (1). It is surprising to many physicians that the present strength of the managed health care delivery system had its origins in a congressional bill passed in the early 1970s. The purpose of that legislation was to stimulate the number of covered lives (people receiving their health care by a managed care plan) in this country and to increase the number of HMOs. Before discussing this important federal law further, we shall review the status of managed care in this country prior to its passage.

The origins of managed health care in this country go back to the early 1900s, when medical services and hospitalization were provided to railroad workers for a specified time period for a specific amount of money. The first "prepaid group practice" (PPGP), the Ross-Loos Clinic in Los Angeles, was founded in late 1920s to provide health services to the city's water workers (2). The clinic was paid a monthly fee in advance for the care. The Kaiser-Permante Group practice and the Group Health Cooperative of Puget Sound were formed shortly thereafter as PPGPs. PPGPs included a physician group providing care in a single facility with a common medical record. The patients were prepaid members, employees and dependents of employers who purchased the health care coverage. The PPGPs were able to convince the employers to offer both traditional indemnity and prepaid health care coverage to their employees. The origins of the open enrollment period offered to today's employees date back to the early 1950s, when the decision was made to offer employees a choice between the traditional health care indemnity insurance or a prepaid group health coverage (2).

The success of the PPGPs rested with the provision of full health coverage, including preventative services as well as baby care, immunizations, and periodic adult examinations. The accessibility of complete coverage at a single medical group was the attractive feature to employees. It was less important that there were no additional health care payments. These early PPGPs quickly realized the need to observe physician performance as it related to cost of care. Care was provided in an educational environment where decisions were made to provide the most appropriate care in the most cost-effective location. The more service provided, the less profit available to the group. The birth of utilization review can be traced to these pioneering medical groups. When the care provided by traditional fee-for-service insurance plans was compared with that provided by PPGPs, the group practices consistently demonstrated a lower hospitalization rate, lower total cost, and better accessibility of care. Soon, local and state governments were offering these plans as choices for their employees.

The Nixon administration supported the HMO Act of 1973 to address what they considered growing crises in both the cost and the distribution of health care services. President Nixon's advisors on health care included Paul Ellwood, Walter McClure, and Alain Enthoven (3). The federal mandate provided loans and grants for the feasibility study, development, and initial operations of health maintenance plans that could meet federal qualifications. Another caveat of the legislation was that federally qualified plans would have to be offered by employers with more than 25 employees. The available federal funding fueled an unprecedented wave of HMO development in the late 1970s and early 1980s. By 1980, about 5% of all Americans were enrolled in an HMO (4).

The continued growth in the managed care market of the 1980s reflected the desire of American businesses to gain control over and lower their health care costs. The historical fact that health care costs have increased faster than the consumer price index (C.P.I.) in this decade is well documented (5). It was not uncommon for the health care cost increases to be two to three times the annual C.P.I. increases. The manufacturing industry seized this opportunity to offer competitive health maintenance plans to their employees to reduce their overall costs and become competitive in the international marketplace.

At this time, the large national insurance companies such as Prudential, Aetna, and Cigna entered into the health care delivery arena by intensifying their purchases or development of HMOs. These insurance company–based health maintenance plans gained increased market share in many health care delivery markets. The large national insurance health programs were attractive to the business community because of their prior experience in the provision of health insurance coverage and their regional or national provision of service. In addition, the large national insurers gave businesses one-stop health plan shopping by offering a traditional indemnity health plan, a health maintenance option, and preferred providers organizations (PPOs). The advantages included having only one account representative, one monthly premium bill, and one enrollment reconciliation. The employee benefits were designed to encourage employees to shift from higher-cost indemnity plans to the fully funded HMO coverage.

In the early 1980s, preferred provider organizations (PPOs) appeared in the managed care marketplace. A California law abolished the previous prohibition on selective contracting with providers, thus allowing the development of preferred provider health insurance (PPI) that was delivered through approved or participating PPOs (4). PPI was attractive to the consumer because it provided more extensive coverage if services were rendered by a provider under contract with the insurer. PPI was attractive to health care providers because it steered additional patients to the provider for compliance with the plan's authorization procedures and a reduced fee-for-service payment schedule.

The PPO concept has developed new variations. The first was an exclusive provider organization (EPO)—a PPO without coverage for services provided by providers outside the organization (6). Another was the physician-hospital organization (PHO), which was developed to offer discounted services directly to employers, insurance companies, or HMOs for either a full spectrum of service or specialty services or diagnostic studies that meet certain utilization review criteria. The success of the PPO is reflected by the fact that in 1992, an estimated 122 million people were eligible to use a PPO as part of an employer's health benefit plan, and about 38 million workers received worker's compensation coverage through a PPO, according to data compiled from a survey endorsed by the national organization representing PPOs (7).

Another type of managed care plan is the point of service (POS) variety. This type of coverage differs from a PPO in that the basic plan is an HMO, not a traditional indemnity plan. A POS allows the employee to function within an HMO environment with a primary "gatekeeper" yet allows the utilization of nonparticipating providers on occasion at a higher cost to the enrollee. This type of health maintenance plan is the fastest growing in the managed care industry (8). It has helped many purchasers of health care insurance to make the transition from the typical indemnity health insurance coverage to a pure HMO coverage; industry data on POS plan utilization show 65–85% health maintenance usage (8).

What is the difference between managed care and managed competition? The concept of managed competition combines market forces and governmental regulation to reform the health care delivery system. Its leading proponents are the members of the Jackson Hole Group, which include Paul Ellwood, Walter McClure, and Alain Enthoven. This concept of managed competition was the basis for President Clinton's Health Security Act (9). The essential principles of managed competition in health care are universal health care coverage, a federal health care board with oversight responsibility for defining health benefit coverage, establishment of standards for health plan purchasing cooperatives and approved health plans, and defined standards for health outcomes reporting. The goal of managed competition is to empower people, regardless of income, to select their health care coverage on the basis of informed decisions and individual priorities. For the managed competition concept to succeed, there must be a national standard information system that allows comparison of clinical outcomes data. Unfortunately, such a system can only be dreamed of presently.

Managed competition in health care would create a more centralized control of health care with its attendant cost and loss of state authority to control local health care costs. The election results in November 1994 would indicate that the American people want less federal government involvement, more state control, and more market-driven choices in the services they receive. The election mandate of November 1994 would indicate that enactment of managed-competition health care legislation in the near future is unlikely.

A maturing managed care market progresses through various stages. Among the many studies on this progression, the one conducted by the University Hospital Consortium was one of the most thorough (10). Their findings indicated that stage one, or the "unstructured stage," was characterized by employers starting to cope with the increased cost of group health insurance. Initially, employers will limit the benefit coverage and increase the employee contribution or copayments. Commonly, several employer groups may begin discussing coalitions to maximize their health-benefit dollar. It is at this preliminary stage that employers offer managed care health plans for the first time. From the consumer point of view, this state is characterized by the younger employees' enrollment in HMOs.

The impact of stage one on health care providers is that physicians begin to experience a decline in income growth. Physicians who had refused to participate in managed care programs previously now begin to sign HMO agreements. Stage one highlights to the practitioners the complexity of the managed care contracts and they begin to experience the administrative and practice complexities associated with these agreements. Because the providers do not trust the administration of the HMOs, they attempt to bond together loosely in an independent provider association (IPA) to negotiate with these HMOs. The practitioners sense the eventual need to relinquish their practice independence and join a group of physicians to be successful in this type of market. Hospitals and other health care provision institutions begin contracting with HMOs to gain market share. At this stage, hospitals and physicians act independently in their approach to the managed care organizations.

The second stage is known as the "loose framework stage." The managed care companies try to secure additional market share by expanding their provider networks. Their pricing structure tends to be 10–15 times lower than traditional indemnity health care insurance, so employers not only offer these plans but try to motivate employees to enroll in them, resulting in increased enrollment in the managed care health plans. The consumer learns the difference between the coverage provided by an HMO and a traditional health insurance plan. The primary care gatekeeper becomes a household term, and individuals use the practitioner's office more than the emergency room for health care.

In this stage, physicians realize that their practice of medicine has begun to change dramatically. As enrollment in the managed care plans increases, the specialty physicians are used less by the primary care doctors. This decreased utilization of the specialist begins to directly affect the hospitals in the number of patient days. The decreased use of physicians results in providers forming IPAs to market their services to the HMOs and hospitals. This stage begins to illustrate the cooperation necessary between providers and hospitals for success in the market. PHOs begin to be formed to further competition. Hospitals and physicians begin to provide care for bundled fees or capitated payments. Finally, in stage two of a managed care market, the hospitals begin to consider aligning with one another and to align with or acquire physician groups.

The consolidation stage is the third phase in the progression of penetration of managed care into the health care market. In this stage, employers look to reduce the number of health care plans they offer to reduce their administrative cost and may even move to a single-benefit insurer with multiple health care options. This employer move coupled with the less competitive cost of traditional health care insurance results in continued growth in enrollment in managed care plans. Consumers are becoming familiar with the health maintenance concept of health care and preach the benefits of such coverage. All of these factors result in the emergence of a few large HMOs and PPOs in the marketplace. During this stage, enrollment of both Medicaid and Medicare patients in managed care plans begins.

During the third stage, hospital-integrated systems develop, and hospitals continue to acquire specialists and primary care physicians to establish a network of providers. The managed care organizations common in this stage are the PPO, PHO, and the group practice or health care foundation. Both physician groups and hospitals begin to offer bundled pricing packages and centers-of-excellence contracting. The most important characteristic of the third stage for physicians is the common acceptance of risk contracting or capitated payments by providers. By definition, a capitated payment system exists when a provider accepts a predetermined monthly payment for each member (covered life) in exchange for the guarantee of a full range of previously agreed upon health services, which may or may not be required by the individual. This type of contracting typically increases the primary care practitioner's income, while the specialty provider's income continues to decline. Compared with the initial stage, when predominantly young healthy individuals enroll in the managed care plans, enrollment of both Medicaid and Medicare patients makes the assumption of risk by the primary care practitioners in this stage more challenging.

The fourth and final stage is known as "managed competition." In this phase, the employer and consumers begin to make decisions about managed care plans on the basis of quality, patient satisfaction, and outcome measurement data along with cost information. Typically, in this stage, the larger managed care plans have more sophisticated data to use during the enrollment periods, which tends to force the smaller HMOs to merge, be acquired, or cease to operate. The consumer is more knowledgeable and sophisticated about managed care and the clinical results of the available HMOs.

This final stage is a critical time for physicians and hospitals. The various types of collaborations between the two provider groups seek to increase their provider base by merging larger physician groups to be competitive with the larger managed care plans or be acquired by them. With the continued decrease in utilization of specialists and hospital days, hospitals begin to close or change their focus to rehabilitation care or extended nursing care. The excess of specialists creates the need for specialist retraining programs for primary care medicine, which are sponsored by the managed care plans. The successful hospitals tend to be part of a larger health care systems that offer a full spectrum of health care services to large managed care plans under full-risk agreements. Some physician organizations (IPAs, PPOs, PHOs) that have not been acquired by the larger health care systems or managed care plan companies fail. The information system requirements of the larger health care systems or physician groups are to provide consumer information on the quality and cost of care as well as outcome measurements addressing the patient's functional status and well-being.

A review of the large metropolitan health care markets in early 1995 shows cities like Pittsburgh to be in stage one, while Philadelphia, Dallas, and St. Louis are in phase two. The health care markets of Boston, Baltimore, and Chicago closely represent stage three, with the characteristics of phase four being found in the Minneapolis–St. Paul and Los Angeles markets. Practitioners must understand the various stages of managed care penetration in the health care market so they can best position themselves for inclusion.

One of the biggest challenges is understanding the new terms that managed care has brought to the market. Listed below are some of these new terms that are appropriate for managed care health delivery and contracts (11, 12).

DEFINITIONS

Age-sex rating   A process to delineate the provider's capitated payment on the basis of the enrollees' age and disease mix.

Basic health services   All federally qualified HMOs must offer these benefits as defined in Subpart A 110.102 of the Federal HMO Regulations.

Bundle contract   The managed care approach to high-cost health care in which the hospital, surgeon, and other consultant's services are covered under one flat rate paid by the managed care plan.

Capitation   The monthly per covered life physician payment for providing a specific health benefit package to a defined group for a specified time period. The monthly payment is the same regardless of the amount of health care service provided.

Carve out   The assignment by a managed care health plan for the provision of a specific subset of health care services (psychiatric, rehabilitation) to a separate provider group.

Closed panel   Specific health care services are delivered for a managed care company by a an exclusive group of physicians, and no coverage is available outside that group.

Contract mix   The description of enrollees assigned by contract to a provider, with enrollees classified as either single individuals, pairs, or families and/or by age and sex.

Covered lives   The individuals that will receive health care benefits from a specific managed care plan or plan risk pool.

Credentialing requirement   A clause in contracts with PPOs that sets predetermined objective criteria for the selection and termination of participating physicians.

Experience rating   The establishment of health care premiums on the basis of a review of actual health care costs for a group.

Hold harmless clause   The segment of a contractual agreement between an HMO and a provider that prevents the provider from billing members for care provided in case the HMO becomes insolvent, denies care, or does not pay the provider's full fee.

Market share   The percentage of the total health care market that enrolled with a particular medical group or HMO.

Medical loss ratio   A comparison of the cost of health care provided to the revenue a plan receives for provision of the care.

Member month   A volume measurement used to express HMO coverage for one enrollee for 1 month of covered benefits.

Open enrollment period   The time allocated for enrollment of individuals by HMOs as part of their marketing strategy. The open enrollment period for federally qualified HMOs must be at least 30 days per year and meet specific federal guidelines to avoid adverse selection.

Open panel   A managed care health plan that contracts with physicians to provide care in their offices.

Par provider   A physician or other health care provider participating in a managed health care plan.

Physician practice appraisal   The audit of a practice according to standards a managed care plan sets for providers, which address patient management, productivity, dependability, and attitude.

Per member per month   The cost of each covered life for 1 month.

Per thousand members per year   An indicator of the members' use of a managed care company's services; for example, the number of days per 1000 or admissions per thousand.

Progressive rates   A method of physician payment by managed care companies that implements new capitated rates for enrollees throughout a 12-month period rather than a single payment adjustment every year.

Reinsurance   An insurance purchased by either an HMO or physician provider for specific protection from risk associated with stop-loss or out-of-area health coverage.

Risk   Acceptance of the possibility of financial gain or loss for providing health care benefits for an HMO enrollee at a capitated rate.

Spend-down case   A member of an HMO who has catastrophic medical expenses.

Stop-loss insurance   An underwriting policy that offers protection to an HMO or providers for the provision of health care above a specified limit on an annual basis.

Withhold   Keep a percentage of the annual payment to a practitioner until the cost of the care has been determined. The amount of money returned to the provider is determined by previously agreed upon utilization rates, quality indicators being met, or a specific satisfaction level being achieved.

REFERENCES

1. Nelson J. The history and spirit of the HMO movement: the early years. HMO Pract 1987;1:75–85.
2. Volpe FJ. Types of managed health care organizations. In: Bloomberg MA, Mohlie SP, eds. Physicians in managed care. Fredericksburg, VA: Bookcrafters, 1994:7–26.
3. Ellwood PM. Health maintenance strategy. Med Care 1971;May:250–256.
4. Enthoven AC. The history and principles of managed competition. Health Affairs 1993;12(s):24–48.
5. Domolky S. Health care reform and the practice of medicine. Med Staff Counselor 1993;7: 1–17.
6. Wagner ER. Types of managed care organizations. In: Kongstvedt PR, ed. The managed health care handbook. Gaithersburg, MD: Aspen 1993:12–21.
7. SMG Marketing Group. American Association of Preferred Providers Organizations Survey. Marion Merrell Dow Managed Care Digest, PPO ed., 1993.
8. Group model HMOs make biggest gains through use of POS products. Managed Care Outlook 1994;7:1–2.
9. Stenholm CW. Managed competition: a health reform plan that "puts people first." J Am Health Policy 1993;1:15–18.
10. Managed care network development: models and tactics for academic health centers. Oak Brook, IL: University Hospital Consortium, January 1995.
11. Managed care comes of age. A glossary of terms. Med Group Manage J 1993;40:96, 98, 100–102.
12. A glossary of managed care terms. Tampa: American College of Physician Executives, 1993.

SECTION TWO

MANAGED CARE REIMBURSEMENT

□

CHAPTER FOUR

PRIMARY CARE AND SPECIALTY REIMBURSEMENT

Judy Harrington and J. Thomas Danzi

As the penetration of managed care increases in a local health care market, the apprehension and anxiety levels of physicians increase. These feelings often result from their misunderstanding of the payment methodologies that are typical of managed health care plans. The prevalence of these managed care payment myths commonly result in feelings of concern, despair, and uncertainty.

Most physicians in this country have never practiced in a managed care environment and received their formal medical training after World War II, which ushered in the presence of indemnity health insurance. The patient and physician grew accustomed to the freedom of selection of their providers and institutions, with no utilization review of services provided. Under this fee-for-service arrangement, the insurance companies reimbursed health care providers either for charges or on a community rating scale. The more health care services delivered, the more revenue for the providers.

Unfortunately, the health care community has done a very poor job in the past 40 years in documenting the value of the care it provided. There are few meaningful outcome data that health care providers can use to demonstrate the quality and cost effectiveness of the care provided (1). The only data readily available are financial information, which often demonstrates the use of high-cost, high-technology medicine without proven clinical benefit. The major purchasers of health care, governments and employers, have demanded decreased health care costs; therefore, the emergence of the managed health care delivery system (2).

Most active practitioners in this country were trained as the "captain of the ship" and learned few, if any, team-building skills. Students learned to diagnose and treat disease. Suddenly, the paradigm has shifted from treating individuals with diseases to one of teams restoring or maintaining the health of populations (3). Given this shift, it is easy to understand the apprehension and anxiety that many physicians have today as the managed care health delivery system continues to gain market share nationally. This chapter reviews the major types of financial incentives that managed care companies can use to reimburse physicians.

In the early emergence of managed care, providers often continued to be reimbursed under a fee-for-service (FFS) payment schedule. Typically, a managed care company offers a discounted FFS schedule that is based on a discount off the customary charge for that type of provider or a relative value system similar to that of Medicare (4). The discounted FFS may or may not include laboratory tests; one should not assume anything in negotiations with a managed care company. Many managed care companies offer global fees, that is, a single payment for all services related to a specific episode of care or medical procedure. The most common global fee application is for obstetrics, in which a single fee is paid for all prenatal and postnatal visits, the delivery, and ancillary tests. Recently, global fees have been applied to specific surgical procedures, such as arthroscopic knee surgery, which include any operations within 2 years of the original surgery, follow-up visits, and diagnostic tests.

As the market matures and managed care penetration increases, physicians are offered and accept capitated payment schedules (5). Capitation reimburses providers a set amount of money per member per month. This "PM PM" reimbursement is commonly referred to as the capitation rate, or "cap rate." The provider is paid the capitation rate on each member monthly regardless of whether health services are provided or not and regardless of the cost of the services. Capitation payments involve risk sharing by the provider and the managed care company. Thus, the physician is assuming all or part of the risk that insurance companies formerly assumed under the traditional indemnity reimbursement system. The risk may involve the total health care costs for a specified population. This fact shifts the physician's focus from treating individual patients to accepting the responsibility for providing cost-efficient care to a specified group or population (member panel) (6).

The managed care plan profits if it experiences growth and its predicted total health care costs are lower than the actual costs for its members for the year. This is known as the *medical loss ratio*. Both capitated and noncapitated health care costs comprise the total predicted costs for the specified time period; however, the capitated costs are fixed. The physician has the incentive to provide quality, cost-efficient care within the margin established by the capitated rate (7). The total health care cost for the provider's services will be compared with the previously predicted provider cost. Providers who can manage the comprehensive care of their members will benefit or "win" from a capitation arrangement. Aligning incentives through capitation encourages a partnership between the plan and provider, in contrast to the more traditional antagonistic relationships that have existed with the indemnity health coverage agreements.

A primary care physician (PCP) assumes the risk for the provision of needed services by the members selecting his or her member panel. PCPs *must* understand what services are covered in the capitation payment. Services that could be in a PCP's capitated payment include office visits, certain laboratory tests (CBC, urinalyses), and selected diagnostic studies (ECGs or spirometries performed in the office). Some plans include the cost for immunizations and newborn care in the PCP capitated rate; other plans cover these services with a curve-out payment.

A PCP must know whether the contract provides for a capitation adjustment (outlier adjustment) if a member assigned to the patient pool develops a catastrophic illness. Presently, most managed care plans delineate cap rates on the basis of the age and sex of the members in the PCP pool (8). There are new ambulatory-care severity-adjusted systems that will better adjust the risk assignment for a physician's member panel (9). It is important to have separate capitation rates for plans that enroll Medicaid and Medicare patients, because their severity-of-illness index is usually higher.

Presently, most capitation rates for PCPs are calculated on actuarial tables of member usage in a managed care environment. The providers must ensure that the historical data set used by the plan is accurate and reflects the current community ratings for PCPs. If the PCPs are going to be at risk for all services, the capitated rate should consider not only the frequency of visits to the PCP per year (typically 3–4 visits per member per year) but also rates of referral to specialists, the number of hospital days per 1000 members, and emergency room visits per 1000 members. Some health plans have separate risk pools or funds of money to cover emergency department visits, consultative services, and hospitalizations; others include the risk assumptions in the primary capitated rate. The provider *must* understand fully what is assigned to the capitated (at-risk) payment for each member.

The type of practice that the primary care provider has can influence the capitated payment for the physician's assigned members. A pediatrician typically has more member visits per year if the member pool has a large number of newborns with their attendant immunization requirements. There is debate regarding the case mix of primary care internists versus that of family physicians. All PCPs must understand the specifics of the managed care plan's capitation rate.

The arrangements with PCPs may vary, depending on the physician's contracting entity. A PCP member in an IPA or PPO for primary care is likely to have individual physician capitation rates. A PCP who is a member of a group practice or foundation could have both the institution and provider capitated or only the group capitated, with the providers receiving FFS payments. Finally, physicians who are members of a PHO could have both the organization and the individual providers receiving capitated payments. As the health care market matures to level IV, the likelihood of large physician group practices increases. This fact may benefit members of such group practices, in that the utilization review function shifts to the group practice, which can implement its own utilization management philosophy.

What has been the impact of capitation on PCP practice patterns? Capitation forces individual physicians to review their own practice patterns (10, 11). Providers become financially accountable for their medical care decisions. Previously, in the traditional indemnity health insurance scheme, physicians were only responsible for patient care, regardless of the cost. Managed care with capitation makes the physician both responsible and accountable for the delivery of high-quality, cost-efficient medical care (12).

This new relationship between the patient and physician is a major component of the managed health care delivery system. This new partnership between patient and physician can be mutually beneficial. The PCPs who will succeed in a capitated health care delivery system are those who establish partnerships with their patients in exercising their responsibility and authority to deliver cost-efficient, high-quality health care. The health plans must provide their physicians with regular valid information on their quality and cost profiles to provide the necessary incentive to effectively change their medical practice patterns.

Many managed care health plans also offer other types of financial incentive to their capitated physicians, such as withholds, risk pools, or bonus payments (13). The withhold incentive is less common today. The percentage withheld from each PCP capitated rate ranges from 5 to 20%. Return of the withhold depends on the risk-pool performance for that individual provider or a group of providers. There are no published studies to document the impact of withholds on provider behavior. In some markets, the withholds have not been returned to physicians, in part or in total, and thus are viewed as a mechanism for discounting a capitated or FFS agreement.

There is a close relationship between withholds and risk-pool performance that affects actual payments or risk pools (14). By definition, a *risk pool* is an agreed-upon sum derived from a percentage of the plan's premium, from a withhold payment, or from some other combination. The risk-pool funds may represent the payment for members' health care costs not covered by the capitation agreement. There can be a consultative service pool, an emergency room visit pool, a hospitalization pool, and specific care need pools for mental health and rehabilitation medicine. The sums are assigned to these pools on the basis of actuarial calculation.

Quality pools are becoming increasingly popular with managed care health plans. The money assigned to a quality pool is distributed if the physician group performs adequately in regard to the other risk pools alone or in combination, with agreed-upon quality improvement indicators such as patient satisfaction, appointment waiting times, or outcome data. The presence of a quality risk pool is attractive for member enrollment in the plan because it addresses the potential for financially rewarding providers for underutilization of health care services to the members of the plan (15).

Physicians must carefully review the plan's approach to the distribution or risk-pool funds before signing a contract. Are the withholds rewarded on the basis of individual risk pools or group risk pools? If there are aggregated risk pools, how many physicians are in the aggregate pool? Are the risk pools evaluated separately or in combination? Initially, individual risk pools might seem preferable to an aggregated risk pool. However, it takes only 1 patient out of the 250 to 1000 members that a provider may have under capitation to adversely affect that provider's individual performance in regard to the consultative or hospital risk pools. Most experienced capitated PCPs would rather reduce this chance by spreading the risk to an aggregated physician risk pool. Therefore a provider should join a panel of physicians with a history of delivering quality cost-efficient care.

The physician should know whether the pool residuals are evaluated independently or collectively. Is an excess in one risk pool carried over to cover a deficit in another? Would the excess in the consultative pool be used to cover the cost overruns in the hospitalization pool or vice versa? What portion of the residuals left in the risk pools is paid out in a given year to the physician? Does the plan distribute only half to the physicians and carry over the remaining portion to the pools for the next year? Finally, does the plan reward only the physicians with positive utilization records for consultations and hospitalization? All of these factors usually must be negotiated by the physicians with the plan, and each plan has a different approach to risk pools and their relationship to the withhold incentive.

Some health care plans offer bonus payments to the PCPs for meeting agreed-upon performance standards. The standards may be related to utilization rates, quality indicators, or productivity by the provider. As with the risk pools, one must know whether the bonus payments stand alone or are related to risk-pool performance by the individual or the group as a whole.

Another type of financial relationship between the provider (PCP) and the health plan is the concept of risk-limiting threshold protection or stop-loss protection, achieved by purchasing separate insurance. This protects the physician in case an assigned member develops a catastrophic medical illness during the year. Managed care plans have different philosophies regarding reinsurance coverage for the individual provider, and the physician must understand the plan's position before signing a contract. Most plans purchase the insurance as part of their risk assumption, but some plans may want the provider to share some of the cost of stop-loss protection. Some plans designate a specific dollar amount for each member's health care above which further health care costs for that member are not counted against the physician's capitated pool or against the consultative or hospitalization risk pools. Other plans assign a certain percentage of the member's cost above the specified dollar amount against the risk pools. The method of paying for this threshold protection varies; some plans pay for it from the withhold allocation of the physicians, while others assign the cost to the consultative risk pool.

Our discussion has centered on the payment methods for PCPs associated with managed care health plans. What about the specialists? How does capitation differ for specialists providing ancillary services (pathology, radiology) and consultative health care? To date, most managed care plans have not capitated specialists providing consultative health care but have paid FFS according to a plan set-fee schedule. This is starting to change, with some plans capitating specialists and removing the risk funds from the PCP budget (16, 17). It is too early to know the effects of this new arrangement on either PCP or specialist income. Managed care plans have used other reimbursement arrangements with specialists who provide services to plan members. The most common arrangements include discounted FFS, global fees for high-cost or high-volume procedures, and bundled case rates that include reimbursement to a hospital and other physicians participating in the care. The type of reimbursement selected by the plan indicates the appropriate utilization of specialist consultation and high-cost or high-volume procedures.

In contrast, the ancillary services related to the laboratory and pharmacy have typically been capitated by managed care health plans. The plans have benefited from these capitated agreements by knowing in advance the cost of these services, and they can determine the physician-specific utilization patterns. As with physician services, the capitated rates for laboratory and pharmacy services are calculated on an actuarial basis.

Many commercial laboratories appear to be attracted to this type of capitated payment system because it allows them tremendous cash flow advantages for a large locked-in volume.

Enough experience has been gained by physicians to allow comparison of capitation with FFS payments. Capitation provides the PCP with a predictable revenue stream. The income depends upon both the provider's ability to appropriately manage the care of the members in the assigned pool and the mix of patients. Physicians can work collaboratively with the plan's utilization reviewers to maximize their practice efficiency. A capitated physician has incentives to involve the patient and family more meaningfully in health care decision making. Capitation provides an initiative for involving the patient in wellness and health maintenance programs. A capitation payment system removes physician concern about the ability of the patient to pay for their services. In a fully developed capitation payment schedule, the physician's administrative responsibility for billing and collection is reduced, as is the anxiety associated with these functions.

What potential problems exist with a capitated payment system? One obvious concern is the skills required to obtain a satisfactory capitated payment schedule and the ability to negotiate the contract. Some physicians will have to alter their practice patterns and incur new education costs to achieve this change. It will challenge the professional relationships that have developed over years with consultative specialty physicians. There is a concern about the "luck of the draw" in the member's selection of physician. A capitated payment system forces physicians to attempt to assess actual costs per member visit and to increase the profitability of their ambulatory practice by reducing their fixed and variable costs. A perceived concern is the potential to inappropriately underutilize health care resources to increase personal income (19).

The challenge is for the managed care health plans and the providers to meet the obligation of monitoring the quality of care provided and to ensure appropriate utilization of services by documenting the clinical outcomes of its members. One of the major challenges for managed care health plans is to provide consumers with information on the quality of care provided. They must retain members long enough to collect clinical-outcomes data on clinical results and patient functional status and well-being. Most currently available outcomes data address only the cost of care and patient satisfaction (20, 21).

At least one large insurance company, Prudential, has established a clinical research center to address the ability of the company's managed care plan to deliver accountable health care with documentable clinical outcomes (22). We believe that all large, federally qualified, managed care plans should produce accountable measures of the clinical outcomes of the care provided. This would ensure that health care plans provide clinically relevant data on their clinical outcomes to allow members to enroll on a basis other than cost sensitivity and patient satisfaction surveys (23).

Before concluding, we should consider the impact of managed care health plans reimbursement schedules on academic medical centers. There is a growing debate between larger managed care companies and academic medical centers about the responsibility each has in the training and education of health care professionals for the managed care marketplace. Traditionally, the larger national insurance companies have considered that academic medical centers must become cost conscious and cost competitive in the managed care marketplace. Medical school–affiliated hospitals have tended to agree with this premise, but they want the managed care plans to acknowledge the higher severity of illness and case mix intensity of their patients. Many institutions have attempted to develop "centers of excellence" to offer to these health plans on a preferred-provider basis. The cost of educating medical students and residents and the inefficiencies associated with traditional education methods have not allowed the primary care sections to be competitive in the bidding for managed care primary care contracts.

There is general agreement that there are limited dollars available to pay for health care in this country. With the projected reductions in the Medicare funding of medical education and the inability of many medical schools to obtain secure managed care contracts for their primary care sections, where will the funding come from to pay for the training and education of medical students? If indeed, the graduates of medical school will be providing care for the managed care companies in the future, do these large companies have any responsibility for the medical education of physicians and midlevel practitioners? How this question is answered will have a direct impact on the quality of medical education in this country. We believe that all health insurance companies should be required by legislation to participate proportionately in the cost of medical education in this country. They should not only assist the medical schools in changing the curriculum to graduate physicians who are better qualified to succeed in a managed health care delivery system but also financially support the medical schools of this country. For the new health care system to be successful, the academic medical centers and the large insurance companies must cooperate to effectively change medical education so that the graduates—all health care providers—can work effectively within this new paradigm of health care delivery.

In summary, all physicians who enter into a capitated reimbursement agreement with a managed care health plan must take the time to fully understand the contractual arrangements before signing the contract. It would be beneficial to have the contract reviewed by a attorney or a professional colleague with experience in capitated payment schedules.

REFERENCES

1. Ellwood P. Shattuck lecture—outcomes management. N Engl J Med 1988;318:1549–1556.
2. Iglehart JK. Health policy report: physicians and the growth of managed care. N Engl J Med 1994;331:1167–1171.
3. Lolr KN. Outcomes measurement: concepts and questions. Inquiry 1988;25:37–50.
4. Bader B. Capitated payment: how fee-for-service medicine is making the transition. Quality Lett 1993;5:2–12.
5. Vogel DE. An introduction to capitation. Quality Lett 1993;5:13–17.
6. Fitzpatrick WF. Capitation 101: a primer for family physicians. Family Pract Manage 1994;1:47–52.
7. Hillman AL. Health maintenance organization, financial incentives, and physician's judgements. Ann Intern Med 1990;112:891–893.
8. Goldfield NI, Berman H, Collins A, et al. Methods of compensating physicians contracting with managed care organizations. J Ambulatory Care Manage 1992;15:81–92.
9. Horn S, Buckle J, Carver C. The ambulatory severity index. J Ambulatory Care Manage 1988;11:54.
10. Hurley RE, Freund DA, Gage B. Gatekeeping effects on patterns of physician use. J Fam Pract 1991;32:167–174.
11. Hillman A, Pauly MV, Kerstein J. How do financial incentives affect physician's clinical decision and the financial performance of health maintenance organizations. N Engl J Med 1989;321:86–92.
12. Povar G, Moreno J. Hippocrates and the health maintenance organization. Ann Intern Med 1988;109:419–424.
13. Kongstvedt PR. Compensation of primary care physicians in open panels. In: Kongstvedt PR, ed. The managed care handbook. Gaithersburg, MD: Aspen, 1993:55–69.
14. Goldfield NI, Berman H, Collins A, et al. Methods of compensating physicians contracting with managed care organizations. J Ambulatory Care Manage 1992;15:81–92.
15. Povar G, Moreno J. Quality in managed care: prying open the "black boxes." QRB 1991;17:341–383.
16. Lazarovic J. Specialty capitation and effectiveness assessment. Physician Executive 1993;19:32–35.
17. Malcolm CL. Specialty service contracting. Topic Health Care Financ 1993;20:68–75.
18. Mangan D. How one group of specialists is coping with capitation. Med Econ 1994;71:132–134, 36.
19. Vogel DE. The health maintenance organization must focus on maximizing value. Manag Care Q 1994;2:80–82.
20. Smith AE. Get past the current cost focus and concentrate on outcomes. Mod Healthcare 1993;23:32.
21. Retchin SM. The quality of ambulatory care in Medicare health maintenance organizations. Am J Public Health 1990;80:411–415.
22. Roper W. Conducting outcomes research within a provider setting: conflicts and opportunities. 1994 Congress on Health Outcomes and Accountability, Washington, DC, Dec 12, 1994.
23. Deming QB. A prescription for national health care reform. Hosp Pract 1993;28:21,25–28.

CHAPTER FIVE

"AT-RISK" SPECIALTY CONTRACT NEGOTIATIONS

Peter Chodoff and David B. Nash

The United States is reorganizing the 17% of its gross national product it spends on health care. This is part of the largest industry reorganization since the 19th century—the corporatization of American health care (1–3). These changes are occurring because of the demands of the corporate purchasers of health care and not because of legislation from Washington, D.C. All aspects of a physician's professional life will be affected: practice structure, hours, referrals, medical staff organization, oversight by other professionals, and administrative structure.

Three of the most important elements of the emerging health care system are risk sharing, capitation, and vertical integration. One must understand these concepts as they stand alone and how they are related. Large payer groups are concentrating their businesses with large local providers and asking them to share the capitated risk for entire populations. Providers (physicians and smaller independent hospitals) are now afraid of being excluded from participating in these large integrated health care systems and have begun to merge to be able to survive in the new milieu. These changes, vertical integration and capitation, demand that the organization eliminate "turf" issues and replace them with a matrix structure that operates on functional lines. The aim of this chapter is to provide physician specialists with information that will enable them to make an informed decision when joining one of the new health care systems.

HOSPITAL RESPONSE

Beginning with the advent of managed care in the 1970s, some form of capitation is becoming the dominant payment mechanism. Coupled with a seamless vertically integrated health care system, they will be the major instruments in providing cost-effective quality health care. According to a recent study, 54% of HMOs use capitation as a reimbursement method (4), and payers nationwide are pushing this risk-sharing mechanism.

Managed care comes in a variety of models (see "Definitions," below) and is the fastest growing segment of the hospital business (5). Estimates have 80% of the population receiving their health care in this manner by the year 2000. Managed care is transforming the business a hospital is in: the structure of the organization and the location of where its services are provided. Of these changes, capitation is the most important and will be the dominant player in health care reimbursement. Capitation changes everything 180°, including the logic, incentives, and conduct of all the players (3). This requires significant behavioral changes on the part of practicing physicians. One study estimated that 80% of future savings will be realized through modified physician conduct, not greater hospital efficiency. This system will impose on practicing physicians detailed oversight of their processes of care and analysis of their outcomes of care.

Health care organizations must now position themselves to increase the number of covered lives they are responsible for rather than be concerned about the daily census figures for inpatient care. Other changes precipitated by the capitation versus the fee-for-service mind set are

- Lower hospital occupancy equals higher profits
- Fewer patient visits equals higher physician income
- Less care equals higher profits
- Care will move to the outpatient setting
- There will be an emphasis on preventive care
- More capital will be spent on sophisticated information systems
- Management emphasis will be on providing the correct modality of treatment

The shift to capitation means that health care providers share the financial risk in providing care to a defined population and are rewarded financially for eliminating unnecessary care (3). The test for appropriate care is "the right care, the right procedure, in the right setting, in the right amount."

PHYSICIAN RESPONSE

Physicians will be required to share in all of the decisions of the vertically integrated health care system. This requires that physician and hospital administrators function as a seamless team. They will help develop cost-effective, quality care plans that all members of the organization will use. The staff/equity model of vertically integrated systems will shift physician compensation to either a fixed salary or salary plus incentive system. Either one of these payment schemes will mean that the revenue streams for the entire organization will merge. This makes the physician dependent on the financial well-being of the entire organization. Specialists are particularly at risk. Their incomes, power, and prestige will diminish.

Clinical practice guidelines (CPGs) have been developed to reduce unexplained variation in clinical practice, provide cost-efficient care, and produce better outcomes (6). Many fully integrated systems contracting with managed care organizations are requiring the use of CPGs. This will limit the number of consultations and transfer some specialty procedures to the primary care physician. Physicians need to be involved in each organization with the development of CPGs so that they have a sense of ownership of the CPG (7).

Part of the transformation taking place in health care is in evaluating the quality of care delivered (8). There is a change from the traditional quality assurance (QA) search for the "bad apple" to continuous quality improvement (CQI) that looks at systemwide processes. Ancillary personnel will play a larger role in monitoring and delivering care. This is particularly true in the home health care segment. The role of physicians in the CQI process is problematic, since many physicians have been taught to think of themselves as independent practitioners and not part of a complex systematic process (9). The first of many behavioral changes required of physicians is their willingness to realize they are dependent on these systems for their ability to produce health care benefits. Specialist physicians will have to learn to work with teams and understand the expertise each member of the group brings to the process (10, 11). Some organizations have found it easier to get generalist physicians to accept this concept than specialist physicians (9). This will mandate that specialist physicians accept a broader role in any new health care system they join. All of these changes will demand that individual practitioners change their focus from intradepartmental activity to systemwide interdepartmental activity.

DEFINITIONS

The following items will come up repeatedly in discussions you will have regarding working conditions. They will appear in contracts you will sign. You must understand what they mean to your professional and financial well-being (12, 13).

Vertically integrated system   A seamless connection among all the elements in a health care system. This includes acute care, preventive care, rehabilitative care, outpatient care, home care, and hospice care.

It enables the institution to change the modality and site of care without regard to reimbursement.

Managed care network   A vertically integrated health care system in which providers and facilities care for a defined population, in a geographically described area, who are in all phases of health. Health is categorized broadly as health promotion to hospice care, including everything in between.

Capitation   Payment for what is expected to be provided. It is a prospective payment method based on an actuarial projection of utilization rates and service benefits for a defined population. (See section on capitation, below.) This will become the dominant form of reimbursement.

Capitation calculation   The product of usage (utilization) of services times the cost for each of these services for a given period, usually expressed as cost per member per month ($PMPM). Accurate and relevant data are necessary for this calculation. Information about the population to be covered is necessary including, age, sex, life style, type of employment. This is part of the concept of risk adjusting, which in this context is population-based compared with severity-of-illness adjustments used on individual patients.

Global capitated system   A system in which the provider, usually a physician-hospital organization (PHO) or hospital, takes one capitation payment covering all services, then pays other providers. Since the globally capitated provider controls the entire system's revenue stream, it can capture the savings of capitation.

Typical capitated system   An insurance company or HMO sets separate capitation rates for different services. The insurer controls the revenues and can capture most of the savings of capitation.

Fee-for-service   Payment for a service rendered in the past for an eligible person or paid for out-of-pocket by purchasers of care. Fee-for-service is payment for what was provided. This type of reimbursement will decrease.

Clinical practice guidelines   Systematically developed statements to assist practitioners and patients about appropriate health care for specific clinical circumstances. They have been designed as one tool to help reduce unexplained variation in clinical practice, control costs, and produce better patient outcomes. In organizations that share risk with the purchasers of care, the use of clinical practice guidelines is a prominent part of their delivery system.

Critical pathways   Locally developed hospital-specific detailed patient-management plans for a particular condition or procedure. They include all the health care providers involved and hospital administrative functions.

Solvency requirements   Any organization that offers health care on a capitated basis is in effect becoming an insurance agency and needs to have adequate financial reserves to ensure solvency.

Risk adjustment   In the capitated environment, a population-based analysis for characteristics that influence utilization.

Stop/loss   Expenses over a set amount are not charged to the provider but are paid for by the plan or reinsurer. It usually is in the form of insurance coverage taken out by a plan to provide protection from losses resulting from claims greater than a specific dollar amount per covered person per year.

Withhold   A certain percentage of capitated payment to cover deficit of another provider.

Medical loss ratio (14)   The cost of medical services as a percentage of the revenue from premiums. Another way of describing it is the number of services a plan's physicians and other health care professionals provide to enrolled patients weighed against the plan's available resources.

Point of service (POS)   A benefit program in which customers receive higher benefit levels when care is obtained in network than when care is obtained out of network.

Preferred provider organization (PPO)   A group of physicians and/or hospitals that have agreed to serve members at a discounted fee for service.

Independent practice association (IPA)   A group of physicians loosely organized to manage administrative and practice costs. Each physician retains control over his or her practice.

Bonus   Money paid over the capitated reimbursement rate for meeting predetermined performance criteria. These can be for preventive services, following practice guidelines, controlling utilization, and meeting quality standards.

Case management   Any utilization review or precertification program(s) that require authorization of benefits before or during the rendering of care.

Coinsurance   A payment liability calculated as a percentage of the payment schedule that a customer is required to make to a participating provider for covered services.

Deductible   A specified amount, which the customer is responsible for in a specific period of time for covered services before the managed care plan or insurance will assume liability for all or part of the remaining covered services.

Health maintenance organization (HMO) An entity that provides, offers, or arranges for coverage of designated health services needed by plan members for a fixed prepaid premium.

Adverse selection (15) When an insured (member of defined population) knows more about his or her health status than the insurer or organization (including physicians) paying for the health care can ascertain. It is distinguishable in the following ways:

At time of issue The inherent risk characteristics of the insured are not properly evaluated.

Due to normal lapsation Voluntary lapse of policyholders who are better risks.

CAPITATION

Capitation is such an important part of the new practice environment that we must understand what it is, how it is calculated, and what changes it will mandate in how health care is delivered. Capitation as a form of payment forces providers of care to share the financial risk for populations of patients and radically alters the incentives and conduct of all health care providers, including physicians (3). Under fee-for-service, market share is measured by the number of admissions, number of visits, and number of procedures. Under capitation, market share is measured by the number of covered lives. Costs in a fee-for-service system are measured by cost per procedure and cost per stay. In a capitated system, costs are measured by cost per covered life, the number of inpatient days, and visits per thousand covered lives. Management focus will shift from achieving a high occupancy rate as a measure of performance to having a low occupancy rate with the right care provided by the right procedure in the right setting in the right amount. A good hospital bed is an empty hospital bed!

To develop a competitive capitated rate, the following issues must be addressed:

- Inpatient care must be shifted to outpatient care.
- Specialist care must be shifted to primary care.
- Acute care must be preceded by diagnosis and prevention.
- Clinical and financial databases must be merged and have up-to-date accurate data.
- Meeting the solvency requirements to assure financial viability.
- Plan design: copays, deductibles, coinsurance.
- Capitation description: services included and excluded.
- Population to be covered.

- Adjustments for the number of expected large claims precipitating a stop/loss payment.
- Administrative costs.
- Sensitivity analyses—low and high utilization scenarios.

The successful fully integrated capitated system will have to deal with the following controversial decisions:

- Owning the primary care network.
- Redeploying capital to the primary care network.
- Selecting physicians for inclusion in the system.
- Relocating physicians' practices to achieve geographic distribution.
- Track cost-efficiency and quality.
- Excluding physicians on the basis of cost and/or quality.

The population to be covered needs to include the following information for risk adjustment and avoidance of an adverse selection model. Risk adjustment in this context means population proxies for utilization and is different from the use of severity-of-illness measures used for risk adjustment of individual patients.

- Age/sex
- Early retirees
- Employment characteristics
- Size of the population

Capitation will result in the following changes:

- An oversupply of specialists
- A decrease in specialist's income (greater for those who are locked out of integrated systems than for those who are locked in)
- Consolidation of specialty centers

It is estimated that if 15% of the population is covered by capitated systems, annual savings would be 79 billion dollars (4). If this grew to 40% of the population, a reasonable assumption, annual savings would be 210 billion dollars. Depending on the risk-sharing arrangement, providers may pocket 50% of the savings.

Physician specialists have to respond to these changes differently than primary care physicians (PCPs) do. A physician specialist will have to

- Accept a less prestigious role in the integrated health care system
- Avoid unnecessary expensive procedures
- Accept a more balanced reimbursement scheme in which the PCPs income increases and the specialists income decreases

- Lobby for a system in which referrals to specialists have fewer gates to go through
- Lobby for a sophisticated outcome-measurement system comparing PCP and specialist care
- Participate in the development of CPGs for specialist areas of practice that are being managed by PCPs

A recent study reported that the treatment of depression by PCPs was initially cheaper than that provided by psychiatrists but led to poorer long-term outcomes (16). One of the solutions proposed for dealing with this problem was the use of expert guidelines developed by the appropriate specialist. Specialist physicians should push for reimbursement for the development of CPGs, and they should participate in the monitoring of their use by PCPs.

SYSTEMS

There are five distinguishing attributes of future health care systems:

1. Vertical integration—payees contract with one party for a broad continuum of care: doctors, hospitals, home health care, prevention, and rehabilitation services in a seamless system. There is freedom to reassign patients without fear of revenue loss to the appropriate modality: hospital, surgicenter, physician office, days hospital, home care. There is freedom to alter treatment without fear of revenue loss: surgical, medical, other intervention.
2. Geographic coverage—offers access across a whole city or region. Moves away from the "local community" service paradigm. This enables one employer to sign a contract with one system.
3. Capitation—the provider system itself is at risk for the whole of a patient's care in dollars per member per month ($PMPM) for whatever care required in the appropriate setting. This includes administration, mobile services, outpatient surgery, outpatient medicine, integrated medical campuses, acute care, home health, durable medical equipment, senior care, long-term care, retirement center, and hospice care.
4. Total care per covered lives is provided at a low or lowest cost.
5. Quality—in a fully integrated system, the selection of staff, adoption of practice guidelines, continuous quality improvement, and the use of practice standards is consistently accomplished.

It is important to understand the relationship of a seamless, integrated health care system to capitation and risk sharing as a form of payment. A fully integrated system provides the purchaser of care with an across-the-board menu of services. These include preventive, outpatient, inpatient, primary, specialist's services, home health, and hospice care. To make this array of services cost-effective, there must be risk sharing by all elements of the system. Capitation is the financial method of payment that accomplishes this and forces physicians to allocate resources and services in a cost-effective way. This is a major change in the role most physicians are used to, that is, being the patient's advocate and doing everything regardless of cost.

The major types of systems are (3)

1. Management service bureau (MSO): Physicians purchase practice services from a hospital subsidiary and retain complete clinical and financial autonomy from the health system.
2. Group practice without walls (GPWW): Independent physicians form a loose alliance to share overhead costs and negotiate payer contracts.
3. Open physician-hospital organization (PHO): Joint PHO open to all medical staff members. It negotiates contracts for the group. Physicians retain 100% ownership of practice. Not all of physician income comes from PHO. PHO acts like an insurer and has financial solvency requirements.
4. Closed physician-hospital organization (PHO): Same as above except membership is offered to a select group of high-quality, cost-effective physicians.
5. Foundation model (FM): Health system purchases physician practices under foundation structure, a not-for-profit, wholly owned subsidiary of the system. Physicians remain employees of a separate professional corporation but sign professional services agreements with foundation.
6. Staff model (SM): Physicians are direct employees of the not-for-profit health system.
7. Equity model (EM): Physicians are owners of the for-profit health system.

ISSUES TO CONSIDER

When joining a managed care organization, the specialist physician must understand risk sharing. This requires understanding the following issues and obtaining answers to the questions asked.

- Primary Care Physician—How is primary care defined? Is the PCP a gatekeeper who controls all specialty referrals? Is any self-referral permitted? Some plans permit this.
- Age and sex have been used for a long time for predicting large group utilization. They don't work well for an individual specialty

provider's behavior. How has the defined population been risk adjusted for use of specialist services? Other issues such as employment characteristics, number of retirees, and size of the population should be considered. Are the capitated services well defined? What is offered and what is excluded?

- PCP dumping—When the capitated PCP refers all services to the specialist. Does the managed care system guard against this?
- Physician report card (17)—This will include such measures as the percentage of generic prescriptions written, attendance at internal meetings, percentage of unnecessary inpatient days, member satisfaction, and (for PCPs) preventative services appropriate and offered. Report cards for specialists are being developed by managed care organizations and state agencies. In Pennsylvania, the Health Care Cost Containment Council was created by the legislature to make information available to purchasers of care on the mortality, morbidity, and resource use of individual providers. The intent was to have informed consumers. U.S. Healthcare has a wholly owned subsidiary, U.S. Quality Algorithms (USQA), that has developed a physician report card that it uses in its marketing efforts. United Healthcare (18) in Minnesota has developed a report card with items such as

- Patient satisfaction based on the physician's explanation of care, waiting time, and scheduling
- Infection rates
- Severity-adjusted mortality and morbidity rates
- Patient functional health status scores

The specialist physician needs to know who reviews the individual provider, what the review criteria are, and what the consequences of an unsatisfactory report are.

- What are the stop/loss provisions? How is it provided for? Do losses carry forward to the next year?
- Does the provider have the ability to control utilization? If so, are they reasonable provisions that will not exclude those needing care?
- Are there credible data for determining the predictability of utilization? One needs to review the assumption used in predicting resource use.
- Are guidelines or treatment algorithms used by the plan? If so, does the individual physician have an input in creating the guidelines? It is not fair to expect physicians to use guidelines without

trials of their own and positive feedback regarding patient outcomes.

- PCP services are easy to capitate; specialists are difficult to capitate. Does the plan pay or capitate by CPT-4 code and not by specialist doing the procedure; for example, endoscopy done by Family Medicine, Internal Medicine, or Gastroenterology?
- Capitation will force the PCPs to perform more procedures; how many and which ones (19)? Is outcome measured for a service that can be provided by specialists or PCPs? Are PCPs required to use clinical practice guidelines for specialist-type care? This is important to ensure that quality is not sacrificed for cost savings.
- The party that controls the premium dollar will profit the most. Who controls it and do you have any say in how it is allocated?
- How does the plan measure quality to prevent undertreatment and unduly limited access to necessary care? Have the principles and tools of CQI been introduced into the system? Is the organization's senior management committed to continuous quality improvement?
- How is the managed care system organized? Does it have a point-of-service provision in its plan? Does it have a Medicare and/or Medicaid population in its defined population? If so, how do these segments differ from other aspects of the plan?

SUMMARY

The specialist entering into a contractual obligation with a managed care plan needs a detailed understanding of the system. Although it is difficult to predict the configuration of the health care organization of the future, certain changes appear to be likely:

- Larger vertically integrated health care systems will emerge. There will be more mergers of smaller systems. These will provide a seamless care system with one capitated payment for the purchaser of health care. This means that physicians will change from being exclusively patient advocates to being allocators of resources. The concept of risk sharing mandates this so that the organization can survive financially and provide high-quality care.
- The models in which the physician either works for the system or is one of the owners will dominate. Capitation and the move to vertically integrated systems will require this kind of practice.
- There will remain a small fee-for-service market. It will be difficult in staff-model integrated systems for a physician to have a heterogeneous practice that involves capitation and fee-for-service.

- Quality measurement and analysis will gradually become more important. It will be important for the physician to understand the concepts of continuous quality management, including various care-mix systems. The science of quality measurement must improve to have a significant effect on referrals. Physicians should become more knowledgeable about the various case-mix systems and participate in their use so that appropriate use of specialists will continue. Demonstration of severity-adjusted outcomes with varying degrees of specialist involvement is an example. This will be necessary to protect quality from the tidal wave of cost containment.
- More physicians will work on a salaried basis (7). This is because the staff-model integrated system will become the dominant player in the emerging health care market.
- The physician should understand the risk-adjustment method used to create the capitated rate and be informed about the organization's ability to meet solvency requirements.
- Capitation will become the major reimbursement methodology in the health care system and will require behavioral changes on the part of health care providers.
- Case managers who know the overall treatment plan and coordinate the care on the basis of critical pathways will become more prominent. This means physicians will give up some of their autonomy and be required to work as team members.
- Advanced nurse practitioners will serve as patient educators, monitor patient compliance with treatment protocols, and become more important in the "chronic disease model" of patient care.
- Health care reform will come from the continued pressures on costs provided by managed care firms and from the states, given the new mood in Washington, D.C.
- Research and development will continue to be reduced by pharmaceutical firms as a result of the relentless price-cutting power of managed care buyers.
- There will be a push to change Medicare to a managed care system.
- "Any willing provider legislation" that requires an HMO to contract with any provider willing to work for them will most likely not pass (20).

The delivery of medical care is moving from a fragmented "cottage industry" to a fully vertically integrated seamless system. A paradigm shift is occurring that mandates teamwork, systemwide solutions to problems, and a reduction in the present "turf"-oriented traditional departmental structure (21). Health care organizations will be arranged on a functional basis so they can respond quickly to the rapidly changing health care land-scape. This offers the opportunity to practice better medicine in which pre-ventive services, inpatient, outpatient, home, and hospice care can be dealt with by one payment in one system. Ultimately, a unified health care record will emerge, the opportunity to implement continuous quality im-provement will occur, and physicians may even find themselves working in a more collegial atmosphere.

REFERENCES

1. Advisory Board Company. Vision of the future, 1993.
2. Advisory Board Company. Aligning hospital-physician interests, 1991.
3. Advisory Board Company. Vertical integration strategies for physicians and health sys-tems, 1993.
4. Johnson J, Mitka M. Showdown at capitation corral. AMA News, 15 Aug 1994.
5. Stuart B, Yesalis C. On taking chances with the law of large numbers. Health Services Manage Res 1988;1(3):135–144.
6. Dans DE. Credibility, cookbook medicine and common sense: guidelines and the college. Ann Intern Med 1994;120(11):996–998.
7. Grimshaw JM, Russell IT. Achieving health gain through clinical guidelines. II. Ensur-ing guidelines change medical practice. Quality Health Care 1994;3:45–51.
8. Boland P. Making managed healthcare work: a practical guide to strategies and solu-tions. New York: McGraw-Hill, 1991.
9. Hart J, Coady MM, Halvorson G. The managed care perspective. J Health Admin Educ 1995;1(13):43–66.
10. Nash DB. Overview. In: Nash DB, ed. The physician's guide to managed care. Gaithers-burg, MD: Aspen, 1994:1–11.
11. Katz LA, Cropp MW. Life of the HMO physician. In: Nash DB, ed. The physician's guide to managed care. Gaithersburg, MD: Aspen, 1994:13–29.
12. United Health Care Corporation. A glossary of terms: the language of managed care and organized health care systems. Feb. 1994.
13. Blue Cross & Blue Shield of Delaware. A guide to participating physician group agree-ment. Wilmington, DE: Blue Cross & Blue Shield of Delaware, April 1994.
14. Nash DB. Future practice alternatives in medicine. 2nd ed. HMO practice: advantages and disadvantages. New York: Igaku-Shoin, 1994.
15. Hauloldt RH, Hauser P, Litow ME. Adverse selection in health care. Boston: Millman & Robertson, 1994.
16. Sturm R, Wells KB. How can care for depression become more cost effective. JAMA 1995;273(1);51–58.
17. Berry K. Legislature forum: hedis 2.0; a standardized method to evaluate health plans. J Health Quality 1993;15(6):42.
18. Baskin ST, Shortell SM. Total quality management: needed research on the structural and cultural dimensions of quality improvement in health care organizations. J Health Ad-min Educ 1995;1(13):143–154.
19. Kassirer JP. Academic medical centers under siege. N Engl J Med 1994;331(20):1370–1371.
20. Jarros RK. A perspective on restructuring of health care in the United States. Am Soc Anesthesiol Newslett 1995;2(59):18–22.
21. Rogers MC, Snyderman R, Rogers EL. Cultural and organizational implications of aca-demic managed-care networks. N Engl J Med 1994;331:1374–1377.

□

SECTION THREE

ASSESSMENT OF YOUR PRACTICE FOR THE MANAGED CARE MARKET

CHAPTER SIX

FINANCIAL ASSESSMENT OF PRACTICE

J. Thomas Danzi

The enhanced penetration of managed care in the health care markets across this country is forcing individual practitioners, physicians practicing in a variety of integrated medical group settings, and hospital administrators to reevaluate their budgetary process. This paradigm shift in the reimbursement of health care delivery from the traditional indemnity insurance plans to capitated or risk-sharing agreements has created the need to reconsider how the annual budget and physician compensation are calculated. Most physicians had no formal education in financial management during their medical training. Formerly, a physician or medical group practice was compensated for the amount of services provided. The traditional indemnity health insurance plan was based on production, with the provider receiving payment for the services provided. Under capitation, the plan and providers control the cost of care, and the resulting compensation or income comes from the effective control of the utilization of services and resources.

The vast majority of individual practitioners or small groups of physicians have an accountant on their payroll. The accountant keeps financial records and prepares financial statements for them. A few providers practicing under the traditional fee-for-service payment system used an accountant to address the budgetary and cost accounting aspects of their practices. The accountant was invaluable in the preparation of tax statements and cash-flow statements, but most providers lacked a good understanding of their average cost per patient visit or an effective budget-reporting system to track their fixed and variable costs. Indeed, the finance departmental function provided by larger group practices attracted many physicians to join group practices in the 1970s and 1980s. The group provided the physician with a fixed income that was productivity based and assumed the financial and budgetary functions for the provider.

This chapter reviews budgetary planning and cost accounting to help practitioners understand their historical office costs and their utilization of service costs. This will serve as a basis for understanding what is a fair capitated-payment schedule. This type of information can help the provider make the changes in medical management that are necessary for success in a risk-sharing agreement.

Three areas of accounting are most pertinent to health care: *financial accounting,* which relates to the record keeping and preparation of financial statements; *managerial accounting,* and *cost accounting.* The financial accountant collects dollar data through bookkeeping for the physician's practice. The resultant financial history describes the medical practice in terms of revenue and expenses. The traditional fee-for-service health care delivery system frequently uses a system known as *accrual accounting.* In accrual accounting, revenue value is placed with the provision of services and reimbursement for that service is assumed. The accrual accounting methodology can also recognize the expense or cost of the service.

The specific guidelines or rules that govern the financial accounting process are known as the *generally accepted accounting principles* (GAAP) (1). As with any profession, accountants vary in their compliance with these guidelines as they relate to specific ledger entries. An external review of your accountant's representation of the financial data by a certified public accountant (CPA) verifies compliance with the GAAP. The CPA's statement will attest to the validity of your accountant's financial statements.

Accurate financial statements are of valuable assistance in the transition to a capitated-payment schedule. These financial statements in combination with a correlated list of patient visits, case types, and services provided could be the basis for cost accounting, which identifies the costs associated with provision of specific services and the impact that volume will have on those costs.

Expenses or costs described in relation to volume are typically separated into fixed and variable components. By definition, a *fixed cost* is an expense that does not change with the volume of patients served by the practice. Some examples of fixed costs in office practice are the salary of the office receptionist, the lease or rental payment, and liability insurance premiums. A *variable cost* is an expense that usually varies directly with volume. A typical variable cost is the cost of office supplies such as pharmaceuticals. Therefore, the total cost of a service represents the sum of the fixed and variable costs for that service, or the total cost per unit. Health care delivery has a higher percentage of fixed cost relative to total cost than other service industries (2). This highlights the importance of high volumes to offset the higher fixed cost in developing an average total cost per unit of service. Tables 6.1 and 6.2. illustrate that the average variable cost per unit of service is less volume sensitive than the average fixed cost.

Two other important cost-accounting concepts are applicable to the financial assessment of a medical practice in a capitated health care market. The first relates to distinguishing between controllable direct and indirect costs. Direct costs of a patient visit include office supplies and support personnel time (receptionist and nurse); indirect costs of a patient visit include the accountant's salary, billing, liability insurance, and other fixed costs. The distinction between direct and indirect costs is important because one can assign accountability for the control of a certain percentage of these costs. If you can control 95% of your fixed and variable costs, it establishes your profit margin for an office visit at 5%. This same type of cost accounting should be done for all services provided. You should know your profit margins for the performance of specific laboratory tests, ECGs, and such diagnostic procedures as flexible sigmoidoscopy and spirome-

Table 6.1
Fixed and Variable Costs

Fixed costs (annualized)	
Rent or lease	$20,000
Liability insurance	10,000
Depreciation	10,000
Salaries (total)	130,000
Pension	10,000
Benefits	10,000
Taxes	10,000
Subtotal	$200,000
Variable costs (annualized)	
Supplies	$10,000
Telephone	20,000
Advertising	10,000
Subtotal	$40,000
Total cost	$240,000

Table 6.2
Effect of Volume Changes on Average Total Cost

PATIENT OFFICE VISITS	AVG. VARIABLE COST	AVG. FIXED COST	AVG. TOTAL COST
1,000	40	200	204
5,000	8	40	48
10,000	4	20	24

try. Another name for indirect costs is *overhead costs.* These costs are more difficult to control because they are not directly related to the provision of care. Importantly, overhead costs have no direct relationship with revenues. It is difficult to know the correct amount of overhead for a specific amount of revenue; thus these indirect costs are typically shared by each type of service provided.

The second cost-accounting concept, *opportunity cost,* directly relates to the resource-utilization changes that all capitated physicians must make to be successful in risk-sharing agreements. The basic idea is reducing the cost of care provision by selecting a barium enema instead of a diagnostic colonoscopy or performing limited hepatobiliary ultrasound instead of a complete abdominal CT scan. Such changes are of considerable importance with a capitated-payment agreement in which the revenue is fixed and the net income results from controlling costs compared with the product of the capitation rate and the number of members per month assigned to the provider. Obviously, the two factors that control a provider's income in a capitated-payment agreement are the unit cost to deliver a service and the specific utilization of services.

Physicians (or their accountants) can use this type of cost-accounting information to establish the cost per unit service for the services provided in their practice. It is recommended that this type of historical cost accounting use 2–3 years of financial data to establish a reliable benchmark for your cost of various units of service. Depending upon the stage of penetration of managed care in your health care delivery market, these financial data can be used in a bid for a discounted fee-for-service rate in an immature managed care market or in negotiations with a managed care company to establish your capitated rate for your monthly per member reimbursement.

The final area of accounting that is useful is *budgetary accounting.* If you have revenue and expense budgets and know the variance from budget analysis per month, you can understand the historical variances in the budget as they relate to the number of patients treated and the services used. Review of a cash-flow budget will identify the times of the year when there has been excess cash for investment in equipment or income-generating plans.

An important difference between fee-for-service and managed care's capitated-payment schedule is the longevity of the patient-physician relationships (3). The traditional indemnity health insurance coverage tended to foster long-term relationships between a provider and a patient. This helped the practitioner establish a relatively stable budget with certain limitations through the years. The physician had a historical record of new patients who were referred by existing patients or other physicians. Because of managed care's yearly enrollment periods, a practitioner can experience a decrease or an increase in patient visits as enrollment changes. This variability makes it difficult for the provider to accurately budget for the coming year. This fact is especially important for providers in a matured managed care market in which usually more than 75% of a provider's patients are capitated (4). The variability of patient numbers is less important when the managed care patients constitute less than 20% of the total (4).

Accumulating evidence from providers who have made the transition through maturation of a managed care market indicates that once the percentage of capitated patients reaches 50%, most providers want to achieve a 100% capitated-patient base (4). This results from the fact that it is more financially rewarding to practice cost-efficient medicine within a capitated-payment system. The guaranteed monthly payments for patients and the ability to control practice costs and the utilization of services provided commonly results in a higher profit margin than with fee-for-service medical care. The incentives in fee-for-service medicine to perform borderline procedures and have unnecessary visits are not compatible with successful prepaid health care. The key is the provider's ability to understand his or her office costs and control the unit-of-service cost. Physicians who succeed in controlling their practice costs and the utilization of services provided to patients are usually rewarded by the managed care companies through withhold or quality risk-pool arrangements and the assignment of more enrollees for the next year.

Physicians who are members of group practices and have traditionally had their salaries based on a production model within the fee-for-service reimbursement system need a different type of financial assessment. It is difficult for group practices to establish an equitable compensation methodology as the group replaces some or all of its revenues with capitated payments (5, 6). A reimbursement system based on production for the members of the group is not logical after the group's total revenue is more than 50% capitated, because capitation has an inverse relationship to the production philosophy. A simple fixed-salary agreement is not the best option for members of a group practice in a mature managed care market. Incentive payments can be added to a base salary for each physician. This is probably more financially rewarding to the individual practitioners providing cost-effective health care.

No simple income-distribution method is correct for all group practices. The type of group practice will affect the best compensation method to use when most of its revenues are derived from a capitated-payment system. An income distribution system that is applicable to a large primary care medical group is probably inappropriate for a predominantly subspecialty group (7).

Medical group practices that are changing from a predominantly fee-for-service to a capitated-revenue basis must understand and discuss the fundamental differences in income generation between the two reimbursement methods. Without this understanding, the group is likely to be unsuccessful in a managed care health delivery environment because its members will not have made the transition from "production"-based health care to risk-shared health care delivery. Attempting to change the group's income distribution before achieving this understanding will likely mean that the physicians will not accept the new method and the group practice will not be as successful under a capitated-payment plan.

The new *activity-based costing* (ABC) is becoming the preferred method of cost accounting for health care services provided under capitation (8). The advantage of ABC over the traditional total-cost-per-patient method is that ABC takes into account the complexity of office visits and procedures performed and the recognized variability of patients and physicians. This method uses the relative value unit (RVU) concept, which is part of the reimbursement relative value scale (RBRVS) fee schedules. The RVU calculation permits more accurate assignment of the administrative and support costs to each unit of service provided. ABC divides the traditional overhead costs into the four main activities associated with the office practice of medicine: the patient encounter, medical record keeping and scheduling, billing and accounts receivable, and administration. Applying ABC to the previous year's activities allows a provider or a group to compare the actual cost of delivering the health care services with the prevailing capitated rates (9). Thus practices whose revenues were predominantly based on fee-for-service reimbursement can evaluate the implications of capitation income.

For example, Table 6.3 illustrates an appropriate division of salary costs among the four major activities associated with an office practice. All the expense costs should be similarly divided among the four activities; in Table 6.1 these totaled $240,000. Assuming 5000 patient office visits, you can then calculate a cost for each of the four major activities. The patient visits can then be divided into their specific types. The number of office visits, sigmoidoscopy examinations, spirometries and electrocardiograms, and laboratory examinations will each have an ABC established by use of the RVUs for each type of visit or procedure. Table 6.4 illustrates the above calculation.

The activity-based accounting method allows the practitioner or the group to understand their cost for each type of patient visit, brief, intermediate, comprehensive, consultative, or postoperative, based on the relative intensity of the resources used with that type of visit. This method generates a more accurate understanding of the actual, or real, cost asso-

Table 6.3
Salary Expenses by Activity-Based Costing

		DIRECT PATIENT CONTACT	SCHEDULING/ CHARTS	BILLING	ADMINISTRATION
Receptionist	20,000	2,500	4,500	6,000	7,000
Billing clerk	20,000			20,000	
Office manager	30,000		2,000	5,000	23,000
Nurses	60,000	60,000			
Totals	130,000	62,500	6,500	31,000	30,000

Table 6.4
Activity-Based Costing for Visit Calculation

Total patient visits and types	
Office visits	3,000
Sigmoidoscopies	250
ECG/spirometry	250
Laboratory tests	1,500
Total	5,000

RVU-based estimates for types of visits

Type of visit	Number	RVU	Total RVG
Office	3,000	2.0	6,000
Sigmoidoscopy	250	6.0	1,500
ECG/spirometry	250	4.0	1,000
Laboratory studies	1,500	1.0	1,500
Total			10,000

Cost per patient visit = Direct patient care costs + Administration Cost
Total expenses = DPC + Administration cost = Billing = Scheduling/chart
$240,000 = 120,000 + 48,000 + 40,000 + 22,000

ciated with each activity required for a patient encounter. These data can then be used to evaluate the income implications of a specific capitated rate for the practice. Table 6.5 illustrates a contract proposal analysis based upon ABC.

As Table 6.5 shows, the decision to accept a capitation contract requires complete understanding of the costs required to provide the health care services in the office setting. Prior analyzes have assumed that capitation rate applied only to office care of the enrollees and that there were separate risk-pool funds to cover hospitalizations, emergency room visits, consultations, and medications.

The financial analysis of your practice in a managed care market highlights the importance of understanding your profit margins for specific corporate and enrollee volumes. This knowledge is especially important

Table 6.5
Contract Proposal Analysis

Scenario I
  Proposed capitated rate = $5.00 PM
  Enrollee volume = 2000
  Annual revenue = 2000 × 5 × 12 = $120,000
  Annual office costs = $240,000
  Physician compensation is not included in costs
A capitated rate of $5.00 PM PM with 2000 enrollees guarantees a financial loss of $120,000 without including the physician compensation

Scenario II
Proposed capitated rate = $8.50 PM PM
  Enrollee volume = 4000
  Annual revenue = 4000 × 8.50 [× 12 = $408,000
  Physician compensation (primary care physician) = $100,000
  Annual Office costs = $240,000
The positive margin of $68,000 makes this contract attractive

Scenario III
  Proposed capitation rate = $9.75 PM PM
  Enrollee volume = 3000
  Physician compensation = $110,000
  Office costs = $240,000
  Annual revenue = 3000 × 9.75 × 12 = $351,000
  This proposal can be successful with the appropriate utilization of services

in planning the purchase of office equipment while participating in a managed care agreement. Any capital equipment purchases will increase your fixed expenses. Assessing the cost of the new equipment in terms of your profit margin and existing overhead costs is especially important when you are practicing in a fixed-revenue agreement. Many practices realize the need for a new office information system to better manage the cost accounting aspects of the practice. The provider must know if the present fixed expenses will allow a capital expense without reducing the profit margin to an unacceptable level.

Health care provision within a managed care agreement may have a higher administrative overhead for group practices than the traditional fee-for-service health care. The Medical Group Management Association states that the number of nonphysician employees increased from 4.3 for groups not involved with managed care to 5.4 for groups with more than 50% of their revenues from managed care contracts (4). The association explained that the increase resulted from the administrative cost of utilization-of-service review and the cost accounting associated with managed care contracts. These administrative overhead expenses reduce the profit margins for group practices entering into managed health care.

I hope that this chapter provides useful information about accounting requirements for practices entering into managed care contracts. It is imperative that providers understand the actual costs associated with the provision of office care. This knowledge will let physicians analyze managed care contracts from a profit-margin standpoint and control costs to enhance profitability in a managed care environment.

REFERENCES

1. Brealey R, Myers S. Principles of corporate finance. 4th ed. New York: McGraw-Hill, 1991.
2. Long HW, Suver JD. The economics and fiscal management of provider organizations. In: Hammon JL, ed. Fundamentals of medical management. Tampa: Lithocolor, 1993: 83–142.
3. Emanuel EJ, Dubler NN. Preserving the physician-patient relationship in the era or managed care. JAMA 1995;273:323–329.
4. McCally JF. Organizing to manage risk. Integrated Healthcare Rep 1993;May:1–7.
5. McCally JF, Lewis JA, Miskowie A. Capitated income distribution systems: they're better with a new approach. Group Pract J 1994;Sept/Oct:48,50,52.
6. Fitzpatrick WF. Capitation 101: a primer for family physicians. Fam Pract Manage 1994;Mar:47–49.
9. Bodenheimer T, Grumbach K. Reimbursing physicians and hospitals. JAMA 1994;272: 971–977.
10. Yang GY, Wu RC. Strategic costing and ABC. Manage Account 1993;May:33–37.
11. Glennie SC. Activity-based costing. Med Group Manage J 1994;Jul/Aug:88,90,92,96,98.

CHAPTER SEVEN

CLINICAL ASSESSMENT OF PRACTICE

J. Thomas Danzi

Successful physicians practicing in a managed health care delivery system can deliver high-quality cost-efficient care without affecting their patients' satisfaction (1). These physicians have learned the value of appropriate utilization review by the managed care company and proactively participate with the review process (2). They know the importance of enrollee satisfaction with the plan's provisions and the care provided in determining their future patient pool. These providers understand the need to release both plan and physician data to maintain or expand their enrollee pool for the next year.

In contrast, many practitioners making the early transition from fee-for-service to a managed health care delivery system are frustrated by the new review requirements. Frequently, the utilization-review process for both ambulatory and inpatient care is resented. There is skepticism about the need to publish provider-specific information for the plan's members. Some of these physicians cannot make the necessary transition from treating disease to maintaining health, nor do they understand the importance of patient satisfaction in maintaining the plan's enrollment.

Most physicians practicing in a fee-for-service reimbursement environment have never had their provision of ambulatory care assessed. The exceptions may have been members of group practices, but this review was typically not as thorough as that of an HMO. Most practitioners have had some aspects of their inpatient care monitored by the various committees of the medical staff to which they belong. The functions of medical records, utilization review, quality improvement, drug usage, and procedure-monitoring committees are well known to all physicians, but the vast majority have never received information or communication from any of these medical staff monitoring committees because their practice of medicine was within the norm for their group. Traditionally, the monitoring committees of the medical staff did not present diagnosis-specific provision-of-care data unless the physician's care deviated from the peer standards. Thus, most physicians never had data on their inpatient care to demonstrate any improvement in the effectiveness or clinical outcomes.

It is therefore not surprising that many physicians are having some difficulty in adjusting to the impact that managed care has had on their clinical practice. A managed care company uses data to manage health care costs, and the sophistication of the information systems that provide and analyze the data are beyond the common understanding of most physicians who have only practiced fee-for-service medicine. Presentation of their practice data can confuse and irritate physicians until they understand why it is being reviewed with them.

The main goal of this chapter is to help practitioners understand the clinical assessment of their practices that will be the standard in a managed care environment and begin this assessment before the transition. This chapter also describes the new ambulatory patient groups that the Health Care Financing Administration is suppose to be applying to Medicare ambulatory care in late 1995 and their impact on the clinical monitoring of your practice by Medicare carriers.

Initially, the clinical aspect of your practice is most easily assessed in terms of inpatient care. The monitoring committees of your medical staff should have data on your performance. Many hospitals now have physician-specific utilization-management (UM) information that is shared with the practitioners in the performance-improvement program of the institution. Commonly, this utilization-review data addresses the average length of stay and cost per discharge for the most common diagnosis related groups (DRGs) that your department treats. Some UM programs also provide practitioners with data relative to the pharmaceutical and diagnostic study costs. This utilization-of-resources information allows physicians to compare their individual performances in providing care for specific diseases with the benchmark of their peers (3).

Many hospitals have changed to some type of severity-of-illness index to address the common explanation that "my costs are higher because my patients are sicker" (4). Some state agencies are also collecting severity-of-illness data for reports on the comparative performances of the institution's medical staff for selective DRGs. Finally, some states are publishing physician-specific data for either high-cost or high-volume procedures. The availability of such data allows the state agency, institution, and physician to compare providers with the state benchmarks of procedural performance.

The application of different severity-of-illness coding systems have provided an opportunity for physicians to learn the importance of appropriate documentation in the medical records of their evaluation and management of their patients. Frequently, this lesson is learned only after public reporting of unfavorable results by a state agency. The hospital administration should educate their medical staff in the nuances of medical record coding and abstraction to improve report care performance. Another important reason for proper medical record documentation is that the Health Care Finance Administration has recommended that Medicare carriers audit both inpatient and outpatient medical records to confirm that the documentation of the provider's evaluation and management justifies the submitted cost charges. The one assessment that no physician wants is a Medicare fraud audit with its potential fines and resultant loss of ability to participate in the Medicare program if found guilty.

All HMOs want physicians in their panels who do not have a litany of medical record suspensions for failure to comply with medical staff standards for medical record completion or legibility of the record. All payers of health care regard such medical record noncompliance as indicating provision of poor care by the practitioner. The necessity for accurate descriptive medical record progress notes and detailed discharge summaries is obvious to providers practicing in a mature managed care environment.

Another important medical staff function is accomplished by the procedures-monitoring committee. Managed care companies want physicians performing procedures to have excellent appropriateness and effectiveness ratings. A provider does not want a high negative diagnostic rating on procedures they perform, because this could signal a problem with appropriate selection of cases. A physician does not want the procedures-monitoring information to indicate a high conversion rate for selected procedures or a high failure rate in achieving the purpose for the performance of the procedure because this suggests a potential problem with their effectiveness. Finally, the data should show a complication rate within the norm of their local or state peers.

The information that the medical staff monitoring committees have available can be used by managed care companies to evaluate the care you provide in the inpatient setting. Unfortunately for a few providers, these data could be interpreted to mean that their past performance makes them too great a risk to be members of the HMO's physician panel.

Physicians entering into a capitated-payment agreement with a managed care company should realize how much data will be collected on the provision of care for the plan's enrollees (5). Before signing a managed care contract, physicians should understand what information will be collected and how it will be presented. This understanding should allow them to be more cooperative with the managed care company's medical director and benefit more from discussions about the data.

HMOs control health care cost predominantly by lowering the rate of hospital admissions and the use of ancillary services. It should therefore not be surprising that the practice feedback provided by the company will highlight the provider's use of ancillary services (diagnostic and pharmaceutical), specialty consultations, hospital admissions, and emergency departments (5). The utilization review will allow peer comparison of that provider with other providers in the plan. The heightened precertification process for use of risk-pool resources (hospitalization or specialty consultation) by managed care companies educates providers about the appropriateness of their care as well as the appropriateness of the site and the provider of the services (6, 7).

The utilization review by HMOs will assess the provider's use of health promotion and disease prevention techniques. This type of review helps the provider make the transition from the treatment of individuals with disease to the maintenance of health for the plan's enrollees or a specific population.

The assessment of patient satisfaction is another important review tool that most managed care companies share with their providers (9). Most satisfaction questionnaires address the availability and timeliness of appointments, the courtesy of the office staff, and the opportunity to participate in wellness or prevention programs. This type of assessment is new for most physicians making the transition from fee-for-service to capitated health care reimbursement. It presents a new opportunity to learn from your patients how to improve the service you provide.

If the managed care company has clinical guidelines for ambulatory care, another assessment could be your compliance with those guidelines. Noncompliance with the guidelines used by the HMO will have to be well documented. It will be important to validate whether the noncompliance was due to patient or organizational variance. About 50% of the cost of care provided by an HMO is related to treatment of chronic diseases (9). The providers should therefore expect to use guidelines in the treatment of hypertension, diabetes mellitus, congestive heart failure, ischemic heart disease, peripheral vascular disease, peptic ulcer disease, and chronic obstructive lung disease. The goal of these guidelines is to reduce variation in care, standardize resource utilization, and improve clinical outcomes for these chronic diseases while reducing the cost of providing care.

Knowing what clinical parameters most managed care companies use to assess their providers, how can fee-for-service physicians prepare for this type of office practice assessment? The most important step is a self-assessment of how you treat common conditions in the ambulatory setting. This review of your standards of practice will allow you to analyze the resources used in providing care for specific chronic diseases. After your "own" clinical pathway has been established by this review, you can compare your standard of care with known clinical guidelines or parameters published by national organizations as the Agency for Health Care Policy and Research, the Centers for Disease Control, or your national specialty society or those in such medical journals as the Journal of the American Medical Association or the New England Journal of Medicine. This comparison will point out opportunities for enhancing the cost efficiency of care by changing diagnostic studies or pharmaceutical utilization. You can compare your present practice with the guidelines fostered by the managed care company and make the appropriate changes in the way you provide care.

Review of your present standard of care for specific diseases assesses your current specialty consultations, emergency room use, and indications for hospital admission. Sometimes, this self-assessment reveals such dramatic utilization patterns that a practitioner recognizes the need for appropriate changes. Unfortunately, physicians commonly treat specific diseases according to a routine they have used for years; this personal review frequently presents the reality of a need to change their clinical practice.

What about the performance of your office personnel and the waiting times in your current practice? How would your current patients rate your performance on these issues? The questionnaire that a managed care company presents to its enrollees assesses their satisfaction with these aspects of your practice. A physician making the transition to a capitated-payment schedule can benefit from a self-assessment of office functions. Do you know the average time it takes for a patient to get an appointment to see you or the average time that a patient waits in your office to be evaluated? What percentage of patients use an emergency room because of the lengthy waiting time for an appointment? Does your office staff refer patients to an emergency room because of the waiting time to be seen? A physician *must* know this information so that any necessary changes can be implemented before the transition.

How courteous is your office personnel in their relationships with your patients? What is the telephone etiquette for old and new patients? Does your office staff tell patients their expected waiting time to be evaluated? Some physicians know the answers to these questions, others do not. Before making the transition to a capitated-payment agreement, the practitioner must ensure that the office personnel is caring and courteous.

It is commonly stated that the standard for patient visits for primary care physicians within a capitated-payment schedule is one patient every 15 minutes (9). What is your present patient schedule for old and new patients? What is your time for a moderately complex patient to receive a follow-up visit? This assessment of how you regularly evaluate patients is very important. Some physicians will realize the necessity for becoming more time effective in evaluating and managing patients in the office setting. This efficiency of time must not sacrifice the quality of care provided or the ability of the provider to establish meaningful patient rapport (10). Patients must feel that they had enough time with their doctor or they will reflect their concerns on the patient-satisfaction questionnaire. The standards by which physicians and their office personnel are evaluated in the managed care environment have not been previously assessed in the traditional fee-for-service health care market. This represents an opportunity for physicians to assess how they practice medicine and how effectively their office staff perform their functions.

How will the data about your ambulatory practice be presented by the managed care company? Most of these plans address outpatient utilization by reviewing the primary care encounter rates, such as visits per day, percentage of new patients, visits per member per year, and revisit interval rate (11), as well as the ancillary services, prescription, and referral utilization rates per visit. The prescription review could contain information on the number of prescriptions per visit or per member per year, the average cost per prescription, and the percentage use of generic drugs. The referral utilization could be assessed by the number of referrals per 100 primary care visits or per 1000 members per year. There could be comparisons with peers for the cost per referral and specialty costs per member per month. The summary of the data could reflect the average cost per patient visit and the average cost per diagnosis of a specific disease. The managed care plan will present hospital utilization data to the physician that often include days and admissions per 1000 members, the average length of stay, and the average per case cost (11).

The health care plan's medical director will review the data with each primary care provider. If the data show a variance from peers regarding consultation utilization, the review could highlight compliance with the consultative authorization system, compliance with a single-visit-for-consultations policy, and the reason for referral for specific diseases. A discussion about ancillary service utilization could center on adherence to a guideline, consultant's ordering of ancillary services, or the appropriateness of the indication for specific diseases. Finally, a hospitalization rate higher than the peer average could result in a more stringent precertification review, concurrent utilization review, the use of case managers, or a medical director's review.

Primary care providers must fully understand the plan's precertification review process for hospitalization, consultation, and the use of ancillary services. This understanding will allow physicians to change their ambulatory practice to comply. These practice changes could affect your ambulatory utilization rates, but most plans would rather have the resources used in this setting rather than in the inpatient setting.

What are ambulatory patient groups (APGs) and how will they affect your outpatient practice? Simply stated, APGs are the ambulatory care equivalent of the Medicare inpatient DRGs (12). The success that the prospective-payment system had in controlling Medicare hospital cost resulted in Congress mandating that the Health Care Financing Administration (HCFA) develop and implement a prospective payment system for outpatient Medicare health care costs (13). It is somewhat ironic that the success of their DRGs led to an increase in the ambulatory care costs of the Medicare population. Development of an ambulatory case mix system for reimbursement is difficult because of the complexity of the ambulatory care setting. The care provided commonly has a physician evaluation and management component, an ancillary service portion (diagnostic laboratory studies), and a procedural component (ECG, sigmoidoscopy). The challenge is for the ambulatory system to appropriately classify the outpatient visit relative to the resources used. This frequently requires grouping together, or "bundling," services for the ambulatory encounter (12).

The ambulatory patient group developers, 3M Health Systems, recognized the three important components of ambulatory care as patient diagnosis or classification, significant procedure performance, and ancillary services used (14). There are about 300 total APGs recommended, with 145 procedural listings, 72 ancillary-service categories, and 80 diagnostic groups (19). The recommended APGs represent a combination of the ICD-9-CM and CPT-4 codes. The patients in each APG should have similar clinical, resource-utilization, and cost characteristics. While there can be only one primary DRG assigned to a patient hospitalization, there can be more than one APG assigned to an ambulatory care session. To the developer's credit, they recognized that many ambulatory visits are for symptoms such as a headache or back pain, and they assigned patient grouping classifications for the most common symptoms that precipitate an outpatient visit.

The assigned APG will be the basis for reimbursement for services provided and should reflect the intensity of resources used. The new APG classification will assign a procedural listing if it was the main reason for the ambulatory visit; a medical group will be assigned if a visit occurred without a procedure. There will be "packaging," or the inclusion of the ancillary-service cost with specific medical and procedural classifications and discounting of certain procedures because of marginal cost for doing more than one at the same office visit (14). The reimbursement implications of the APGs will be detailed by the Medicare carrier.

Congress charged HCFA with having the APGs implemented by October 1995. It is impossible to state at this time whether they will be compliant with that date. Currently, 3M Health Systems is evaluating the inclusion of patient health status in the APG to determine whether this combination would enhance the ability to determine resource utilization (12). The impact of this research on the proposed implementation date cannot be presently determined, but it is expected to delay it.

The application of the APGs to utilization review will facilitate the process because of the procedural and ancillary service codes. By combining the two prior ambulatory classification methods, the new ambulatory coding system will address the case-mix issue relative to clinical resource utilization in the ambulatory setting (12). This new ambulatory care classification system may facilitate the tracking of clinical resource utilization in the ambulatory setting.

REFERENCES

1. Udvarhelyi I. Comparison of the quality of ambulatory care for fee-for-service and prepaid patients. Ann Intern Med 1991;115:394–400.
2. Franks P. Gatekeeping revisited—protecting patients from over treatment. N Engl J Med 1992;327:424–429.
3. Rosenstein A. Utilization review, health economics, and cost-effective resource management. Quality Assurance Utilization Rev 1991;6:1–2.
4. Kravitz R. Differences in the mix of patients among medical specialties and systems of care. JAMA 1992;267:1617–23.
5. Schlackman N. The impact of managed care on clinical practice. In: Bloomberg MA, Mohlie SR, eds. Physicians in managed care. Fredericksburg, VA: BookCrafters, 1994:27–48.
6. Kongstvedt PR. Controlling hospital utilization. In: Knogstvedt PR, ed. The managed health care handbook. Gaithersburg, MD: Aspen, 1993:102–115.
7. Kongstvedt PR. Controlling referral/consultant utilization. In: Knogstvedt PR, ed. The managed health care handbook. Gaithersburg, MD: Aspen, 1993:116–121.
8. Kongstvedt PR. Formal physician performance evaluation. In: Knogstvedt PR, ed. The managed health care handbook. Gaithersburg, MD: Aspen, 1993:189–199.
9. Knogstvedt PR, ed. The managed health care handbook. Gaithersburg, MD: Aspen, 1993.
10. Emanuel EJ, Dubler NN. Preserving the physician-patient relationship in the era of managed care. JAMA 1995;273:323–329.
11. Kongstvedt PR. Use of data and reports in medical management. In: Knogstvedt PR, ed. The managed health care handbook. Gaithersburg, MD: Aspen, 1993:171–179.
12. Goldfield N. Understanding your managed care practice: the critical role of case mix systems. In: Nash DB, ed. The physician's guide to managed care. Gaithersburg, MD: Aspen, 1994:189–216.
13. Averill R, Goldfield M, McQuire T, et al. Design and development of a prospective payment system for ambulatory care. Final report. Prepared with the support of Health Care Financing Administration, December 1990.
14. Position your program for APG's. Out-patient Reimbursement Manage 1994;1:49–52.

CHAPTER EIGHT

CLINICAL GUIDELINES AND PATHWAYS

J. Thomas Danzi

The health care industry and providers of health care are being challenged to define new mechanisms to ensure the delivery of high-quality, cost-efficient medical care. This demand comes from the payers of health care (health maintenance organizations (HMOS) and insurance companies), the purchasers of health care (employers and employees), regulatory agencies, and both state and federal governments. Success will depend on the ability to better coordinate the care provided, to appropriately utilize clinical resources, to render care in the most efficient time frame and setting, and to incorporate the patient and family into the decision-making process (1, 3). Finally, care provision must result not only in the treatment of disease but in outcomes that address patient functional status, well-being, and satisfaction.

The health care industry is being told to use a variety of standardized care plans, parameters, pathways, or guidelines to achieve this aim (4, 5). These patient care coordinating tools are being heralded as the mechanism for delivery of more consistent, higher-quality, cost-effective health care. The support for the application of clinical guidelines is from the payers and purchasers of health care.

In this competitive health care market and with the increasing penetration of managed health care delivery in the marketplace, providers of health care are using different approaches to enhance their market share. The continuous quality improvement (CQI) philosophy, the patient-focused care ideal, and clinical care coordinating tools are the three main management approaches to changing the methodology of care provision in this country (6, 8).

There are no data to rank these three approaches in terms of their effectiveness or to indicate which is the best method for an academic medical center or a community hospital. The administrative decision is usually based on an assessment of the providers' and management's team-building skills, the institution's empowerment philosophy, and the availability of resources to achieve success with one of these approaches.

Are there essential differences in the three approaches? A close screening of the three reveals a common basis—the review and understanding of the processes involved in the delivery of health care. The premise of CQI is the review of all processes involved in the delivery of health care. The patient-focused care initiative is based on the principle that all health care processes must have the patient's convenience, participation, and satisfaction as the primary goals. The success that providers have in a patient-focused health care environment will be determined by the review of the processes by which care is presently delivered compared with those that will be required. Finally, the development of clinical pathways or guidelines requires review of what care is provided and when and then a description of the proper sequence for the delivery of the care.

Each of these three approaches will require physician participation in multidisciplinary teams that review the processes by which health care is provided. The success of those teams will depend on the ability of the provider administration to have physicians accept a team approach rather than the old "captain of the ship" philosophy. Physicians commonly have weak team-building capabilities. This recognized deficiency must be corrected for any of these methodologies to be successful.

How successful has the medical profession been in developing clinical guidelines or clinical pathways in an attempt to enhance the effectiveness of health care provision? The Institute of Medicine defines practice guidelines as systematically developed statements to help practitioners and patients decide about appropriate health care for specific conditions (9). The payers of health care, especially managed care companies, might define a clinical guideline as a comparison-based standard of diagnostic and treatment modalities for a specific condition. The payer's definition would reflect the patient's participation in the decision-making process, based on health outcomes data. Obviously, the parties involved in the health care delivery system in this country do not agree on a definition of clinical guidelines or pathways. More importantly, there is little evidence for consensus about clinical guidelines in the physician community (10). Some important questions are still unanswered: Is there consistency in the clinical outcomes of care provided by guidelines developed by different physician group analyses of similar clinical conditions? How reliable and valid are guidelines? How can practitioners best become knowledgeable about clinical guidelines?

Two recent articles in the Internal Medicine literature address the American College of Physicians members' familiarity with, confidence in, and attitudes toward guidelines published by their society or other organizations. Tunis et al. found that only 11% were familiar with 2-year-old guidelines published by the college, 7% acknowledged the existence of factitious guidelines, about 80% had confidence in guidelines developed by the college, and nearly 70% felt that guidelines could improve the quality of care provided; but the same percentage felt that guidelines would be used to evaluate physician performance (11). An editorial on this article supported the concept that guidelines should be based on sound evidence and implemented only when data support the health outcomes addressed by the guidelines (12); the author did recommend using the new clinical information systems to increase practitioners' knowledge and use of clinical guidelines.

There is evidence that specialists know more about guidelines developed by their specialty than primary care physicians do about guidelines developed by health advisory organizations (13). However, different physician specialties are defined as primary care practitioners, and no one society addresses their educational requirements.

The Agency for Health Care Policy and Research has been charged by Congress to lead the development of clinical guidelines and determine their effectiveness in health care delivery. This agency has distributed its guidelines mainly through direct mailings to physicians. Unfortunately, there is evidence that such attempted intervention in physician practice style is ineffective, and the agency is presently evaluating its distribution methods (14).

MacDonald and Overhage summarized the physician community's concerns about the validity and reliability of clinical guidelines (15), and provided excellent insight into the challenges faced by the physician community and federal agencies as they develop clinical guidelines. Physicians, as individuals trained in the scientific method, are more likely to change their practice when a guideline is based on proven controlled clinical outcome data.

Before discussing the developmental processes used for clinical guidelines, I would like to discuss the potential impact of physician practice variance as it relates to these clinical practice tools. The release of physician-specific data for comparative purposes has received much attention recently. The customer's need for meaningful information on which to base health plan and physician selection is the major impetus for the release of clinical outcome data. An article by Topol and Califf endorses the provision of physician-specific data (16), while an editorial by Brook addresses the requirements needed before such information should be released to the public (17). It is conceivable that such data could include the practitioner's compliance with clinical guidelines. Since there is no evidence that guidelines define optimal care, it is imperative that comparable outcome data document the validity of guidelines to achieve such outcomes (18–20).

In a classic article, Woolf outlined the methodology available for development of practice guidelines (21). The four methods outlined included informal consensus, formal consensus, evidence-based, and explicit development. The informal consensus method involves expert panels and scientific evidence and results in a recommendation from a specialty society or governmental task force. This method is limited by the validity of using expert opinions as a basis for defining appropriateness. The second developmental process, the formal consensus method, has been used by the National Institute of Health, the AMA, and the RAND Corporation, but the resultant appropriateness scores have little clinical application. Again, the lack of documented outcome evidence means that there is an incomplete basis for the recommendation. Both of these methods can usually result in guidelines being developed within several days.

The Clinical Efficacy Assessment Project of the American College of Physician serves as a model for the evidence-based guideline development process (22). This methodology has been adopted by the American Heart Association and the U.S. Preventative Services Task Force (21). The Agency for Health Care Policy and Research (AHCPR) has adopted this methodology in conjunction with the formal consensus method (23). The explicit guideline development process has gained acceptance by the American Academy of Family Practice and for some guidelines developed by the AHCPR (21). This final process is the most analytical but is probably impractical for clinical pathway development by hospital medical staff. It is therefore not surprising that guidelines for a specific condition that are developed by different methodologies and different organizations often have different recommendations. Indeed, the outcomes predicted by the guidelines could be as different as the analytic processes to evaluate them (24).

What is the best way to implement clinical practice guidelines in either the inpatient or ambulatory setting? I have reviewed the development processes for governmental agencies or national physician societies. Does this methodology apply to development and implementation of clinical guidelines or pathways by hospital medical staffs? Many hospitals have asked specific health care provider teams composed of physicians, nurses, and other support staff to review how care is provided for specific conditions or DRGs. The specific diseases are selected by the hospital administration because of opportunities to improve either the quality or the cost efficiency of care. The cost information usually includes length of stay (LOS) and cost per discharge for the institution, with comparisons available to other regional providers. The quality indicators could contain information from the institution's quality improvement process, with benchmark comparison with comparable institutions. The quality data could result from state-generated comparative data on mortality and morbidity information or readmission rates within 30 days. Usually, such state-published data are severity adjusted for more meaningful comparisons. The best example of state-generated data is that from Pennsylvania's Health Care Cost Containment Council, which uses severity-adjusted data to compare a hospital's projected performance on more than 50 diseases and provider outcome data for coronary artery bypass graft surgery.

The most important part of the developmental process is the selection of members for the multidisciplinary team that will develop the clinical guideline or pathway. It is imperative that respected medical staff and nursing leaders coordinate this process. The data provided to the Advisory Board of Washington, D.C., by its hospital members underscore the importance of pathway team selection. This advisory group recommends that it is better to have leaders coordinate the process and let the skeptics be convinced with its success rather than attempting to convince the doubters to participate in the developmental process (25).

The same consulting company advised that hospitals select only one to five diseases to evaluate at one time. The administration must be able to provide the necessary support regarding disease-specific data and free up the appropriate individuals to participate in the process. Typically, the management team must provide team-building skills for individuals participating in their first multidisciplinary health care provider team. The team members must feel free to say anything without fear of potential retaliation and be able to build on other team members' comments without creating a feeling of insecurity among them.

Many institutions have tried a different developmental process, in view of their physicians' busy schedules. Instead of asking physicians to participate in the developmental process, some hospital administrations have had nurses create the practice guideline or pathways alone. The physician leadership is then asked to evaluate the generated guideline. The advisory board states that this methodology has the highest failure rate for guideline or pathway development (25). Physicians must be involved in the assessment and developmental processes for the clinical pathways or guidelines to be implemented successfully. The American Hospital Association's strategy for clinical guideline development advocates a similar process (26).

Hospital administration must provide the team with existing published guidelines from federal agencies and other institutions. The team members will provide clinical care guidelines from physician and nursing societies. This review process has educational value for the members as they compare the way care is provided at their institution with national guidelines or at benchmark institutions. Identification of one or two new opportunities for enhancing care at the hospital usually signifies success of the project. Explaining the proposed clinical pathway or guideline at medical staff and nursing departmental meetings serves to educate both staffs. The guideline becomes a standard of care for the specific condition at that institution, while the clinical pathway becomes the care-coordinating tool that highlights the critical steps in the provision of care.

Most hospitals that have participated in practice guideline or clinical pathway development have noticed that during the process, the cost indicators commonly report improve. Length of stay typically starts to shorten just because the team is discussing how to enhance the processes by which care is provided. The cost per discharge is usually less during the developmental process but often is positively affected after implementation of the guideline.

One of the main issues that the work team must address is how variances from the proposed clinical guideline or pathway will be assessed. The three main reasons for variances are provider compliance, the ability of the institution's operational systems to provide the service, and the patient's clinical course. The project team must recommend the best method for tracking these variances, and the institution must provide the resources to accomplish the data collection and analysis. The variance data should be reviewed within the institution's quality improvement program so the process is educational and nonpunitive. Without inclusion in the CQI framework, health care providers and institutions will not realize the maximum benefit from development and implementation of clinical guidelines or pathways.

Each institution must recognize how much data variance tracking will produce and the need for appropriate information-system support to manage these data. Without the necessary human resource and information system commitments, the providers and the institution may become frustrated with the process. The Advisory Board refers to this as the "data doom loop process" (25). The provider team member's frustration in trying to proceed without the necessary information can limit the potential of the clinical guideline project; thus the team and the administration must agree on the support required to successfully complete the project.

The public's interest in the application of clinical guidelines is in enhancing the quality of care provided and the resultant clinical outcomes. The developmental process for clinical guidelines tends to address the cost and quality aspects of care without necessarily providing information on the outcomes of the care. Some institutions now ask the work team to assign clinical outcome projections. Planned outcomes should include the patient's functionality, well-being, and satisfaction. If the ultimate goal of this process is to enhance the health of individuals cared for, the emphasis should be on compliance to achieve specific clinical outcomes. Incorporation of clinical outcome goals into the practice guideline developmental process changes the impetus for monitoring and evaluation.

Inclusion of clinical outcome indicators within the clinical guidelines focuses part of the evaluation on the combined efforts of the providers and institution to address the health issues of the patients rather than assessing individuals and individual processes. The public relations value of this is tremendous in today's market, because unfortunately, most institutions do not adequately address the patient's perception after the provision of care. The educational value for the provider's staff in understanding the fundamental paradigm shift in health care delivery from the treatment of disease to the maintenance of health is invaluable.

Implementation of the clinical guidelines or pathways is the next step. It is in this phase that the leaders of the medical, nursing, and ancillary support staffs present the recommended clinical tool for acceptance by their respective staffs. The medical staff endorsement must proceed through the normal medical staff and administrative committee structure. The recommended clinical pathway is then forwarded to either the utilization management or medical staff quality improvement committee for their endorsement and to the medical executive committee.

One important aspect of the medical staff approval process is educating the medical staff about the implementation plan. Will the clinical guideline be first used retrospectively to evaluate how current care provision compares with the guideline or will the guideline be used to provide care concurrently? Do providers have the option of not following the guideline after the implementation date? What data will be monitored on the practitioners and how confidential will that data be? What data, if any, will be shared with the payers of health care? Will the data be used in the credentialing reappointment process for physicians? A successful implementation plan will have addressed these questions before presentation of the plan to the medical staff.

Each component of the health care team—physicians, nurses, and ancillary support personnel—must have a similar evaluation process after implementation of the clinical guideline or pathway. Without such consistency, the maximum benefit from the guideline will not be realized. All monitoring data must be incorporated into the institution's quality improvement process, so that the data are used in an educational manner. All individual information must be kept confidential, and institutional policies should ensure the security of the data.

The work team's responsibility does not end with implementation of the clinical guideline or pathway. This group should coordinate review of the monitoring data to each component of the provider team and to the administration of the institution. Results should be presented at staff meetings, highlighting the impact of the guideline or pathway on accomplishing the predetermined quality, cost, and outcome indicators. Individual provider information should be presented in personal feedback sessions with subsequent follow-up meetings that address predetermined improvement objectives.

The condition-specific work team must reassess the guideline for appropriate changes based on the monitoring information. Teams should not become "married" to the original care plan because this is an evolutionary process. The team members must be told of this aspect of the team's responsibility early in the process. It should be described as part of continuous quality improvement. Individual members should realize that they will not be criticized if the clinical guideline or pathway requires subsequent revision. Rather, the team should believe that they will be successful if this pathway process improves the provision of care.

What evidence exists that the application of clinical guidelines or pathways effects change in the way care is provided? There is little in the medical literature to confirm this impression. A review of the impact of a Canadian guideline relating to cesarean delivery showed that it failed to reduce the rate of cesarean sections 2 years after it had been disseminated to obstetricians (27). The prior release of NIH consensus statements in this country revealed that the direct mailing technique for such guidelines usually failed to produce the desired clinical change unless there were follow-up educational programs (28). These two articles highlight the need for developing and implementing clinical practice guidelines locally rather than at a national level. The local peer influences and the educational value that a successful hospital-derived guideline project affords are the two main reasons for the observed changes in physician practice behavior.

Evidence indicates that the approach most likely to change physician practice patterns is the local hospital developmental process (29). A new economic incentive has appeared in the regional marketplace. Acceptance of physicians into managed care companies will be based in part on their compliance with locally accepted clinical guidelines and pathways (30, 31). The reality of exclusion from a patient source will become the greatest incentive for physicians to change their practice behavior. The publishing of physician-performance report cards in several large metropolitan areas in this country today is another strong incentive for practitioners to practice within locally accepted clinical guidelines (32). Individual physicians who routinely practice outside the parameters of their peers are likely to face both exclusion from managed care company panels in the future and exposure to malpractice litigation. Today's purchasers and payers of health care will not tolerate such previously recognized variances in the performance of procedures or the treatment of disease as outline by Wennberg et al. (33).

There is evidence that regional practice guidelines can enhance the quality and cost efficiency of health care by reducing the number of malpractice claims. If the state board of health requires physicians to practice within guidelines, malpractice insurance premiums can be decreased and the number of malpractice claims reduced (34). Massachusetts requires anesthesiologists to follow guidelines on intraoperative monitoring, and the law states that deviation from the guideline is inadequate and unreasonable provision of care (35). Negligence can be defined on the basis of variance from published recommendations; this is the basis for the State of Maine Medical Association's experiment. This malpractice reform proposal permits physicians who practice within clinical guidelines to use their practice pattern as an affirmative defense that can not be challenged in court (36).

The issue of health care reform and the necessity for tort law reform seem to have a common ground. Some of the high cost of health care in this country has always been attributed to defensive medical practices. The competitive managed care market with its exclusive panels has been an incentive to change this type of medical practice. I believe that without federally legislated malpractice reform, this issue will never be totally eliminated. The federal government should benefit from some innovative state programs that address malpractice reform through the application of clinical guidelines. The issue of the appropriateness of care needs to be directly linked to consensus-derived peer-generated standards of care. Chapter 11.4 in this book discusses the legal aspects of clinical guidelines for physicians and addresses concerns regarding patients who cannot be treated according to the guideline.

The concept of the need for the individualization of care and the practitioners' fear of "cookbook" medicine have changed with the increased penetration of managed health care in the marketplace. Much of the concern about the possible loss of physician autonomy with the application of clinical guidelines or pathways has been reduced by managed care's impact on the need to accommodate to patient preferences that was frequently observed in the fee-for-service delivery system. The public's education has been an important factor in reducing the fear of malpractice claims if the practitioner did not meet the patient's preference for care that was not medically justified. I believe that managed care companies should continue to educate the public about the benefits of applying clinical guidelines (37).

The bioethical implications of practice guidelines for the patient, the provider, and the payers have new significant meaning in this era of health care cost containment. A clinical practice guideline developed at either the national or local level must be compatible with the ethical considerations of all three parties. The physician's ethical considerations include beneficence (promoting good for the patient), nonmaleficence (preventing harm), and respect for patient autonomy in decisions regarding choice of care or lifestyle. The payer's ethical concerns in a managed care delivery model include distributive justice, or the duty to distribute health care resources in a fair, nonarbitrary, equitable manner. The bioethical concerns of patients include autonomy, informed consent, and their ability to make health care decisions.

A newer issue that has gained importance in this highly competitive health care market is the provider and payer's ethical concerns relative to the value of care provided within the financial constraints of the health plan. The Institute of Medicine defined minimum care, and there was concern that such a definition could become a standard for a payer of health care with strong market forces driving the decision process (38). The practitioners worry that care below this standard will become the definition of negligence. It is easy to justify the value of health care provided, but the reality of providing less than maximum-valued care raises ethical questions for physicians and managed care companies. It is currently recommended that clinical practice guidelines not address the minimum-care provision because of the legal and ethical concerns.

A properly designed clinical practice guideline should strengthen the patient-physician relationship and thus enhance patients' decision making about their health care. This clinical tool should help the patient understand the projected outcomes of the care provided and therefore its rationale. The clinical decision-making process should reflect the best interests of the patients while respecting their autonomy.

The Institute of Medicine recommends that clinical practice guidelines address the cost effectiveness of the care to be provided but provide information on the cost implications of alternative care if there is a difference in the quality of life expectancy (38). The reality is that most developers of local guidelines do not have the information to answer those questions. The necessary clinical-outcomes information is not available for most conditions. Therefore, shared decision making between the patient and provider is typically based on legal and/or risk-management values. Guidelines to help the patient understand the risk-benefit ratio of the care provided would be of benefit in a managed care delivery system.

Practice guidelines can also help the patient to understand the differences in the services provided in a managed care plan and an indemnity health plan. The patient needs to understand the insurance plan coverage for immunizations, dialysis therapy, and all types of transplantations. The information could state the various benefits or harm of receiving or not reviewing various therapies or preventive measures, while clearly indicating when there are nonconclusive data on a specific condition. The challenge is to translate the practice guidelines to provide patient information about various therapies and their possible clinical outcomes.

Provision of care according to practice guidelines or clinical pathways will be one factor by which providers are evaluated for inclusion in health insurance plans. The guidelines will represent the health care that providers and payers agree will ensure a high level of quality, appropriateness, and cost efficiency. The author is hopeful that the process outlined in this chapter, the concerns that need to be resolved regarding clinical guidelines, and the bioethical realities of managed care can be addressed successfully, so that these clinical-care coordinating tools can have a positive impact on the provision of health care in this country.

REFERENCES

1. Cordero CE, Christensen L. Practice guidelines are adding value to managed care. Business Health 1992;8:22–27.
2. Kassicer JP. The quality of care and quality of measuring it. N Engl J Med 1993;329:1263–1265.
3. President's Health Care Reform Plan: American Health Security Act of 1993. Washington, DC: Bureau of National Affairs. 13 Sept 13, 1993.
4. Chassin MR. Improving quality of care with practice guidelines. Health Serv Manage 1993;10:40–44.
5. Chassin MR. Standards of care. Inquiry 1988;25:437–453.
6. Greco PJ, Eisenberg JM. Changing physicians practices. N Engl J Med 1993;329:1271–1274.
7. Berwick DM. Continuous improvement as an ideal in health care. N Engl J Med 1989;320:53–56.
8. Lee JG, Clarke RW, Glassford GH. Physicians can benefit from a patient-focus hospital. Physician Exec 1993;19:36–39.
9. Woolf SH. Practice guidelines: a new reality in medicine. I. Recent developments. Arch Intern Med 1990;150:1811–1818.
10. Audet AM, Greenfield S, Field M. Medical practice guidelines: current activities and future directions. Ann Intern Med 1990;113:709–714.
11. Tunis SR, Hayward RSA, Wilson MC, et al. Internist's attitudes about clinical practice guidelines. Ann Intern Med 1994;120:956–963.
12. Dans PE. Credibility, cookbook medicine, and common sense: guidelines and the college. Ann Intern Med 1994;120:966–968.
13. Woolf SH. Practice guidelines: a new reality in medicine. III. Impact on patient care. Arch Intern Med 1993;153:2646–2655.
14. Van Amringe M, Shannon TE. Awareness, assimilation, and adoption: the challenge of effective dissemination and the first AHCPR-sponsored guideline. QRB 1993;18:397–404.
15. McDonald CJ, Overhage JM. Guidelines you can follow and trust. JAMA 1994;271:872–873.

16. Topol EJ, Califf RM. Score and cardiovascular medicine: its impact and future directions. Ann Intern Med 1994;120:65–70.
17. Brook RH. Health care reform is on the way: do we want to compete on quality? Ann Intern Med 1994;120:84–86.
18. Eddy DM. The challenge. JAMA 1990;263:287–290.
19. Eddy DM. Practice policies: where do they come from? JAMA 1990:263:1265, 1269, 1272, 1275.
20. Jacoby I. Evidence and consensus. JAMA 1988;259:3039.
21. Woolf SH. Practice guidelines: a reality in medicine II. Methods of developing guidelines. Arch Intern Med 1992;152:946–952.
22. White LF, Ball IR. The clinical efficacy assessment project of the American College of Physicians. Int J Technol Assess Health Care 1985;1:169–174.
23. Woolf SH. Manual for clinical practice guideline development: a protocol for expert panels convened by the Office of the Forum for Quality and Effectiveness in Health Care. Rockville, MD: Agency for Health Care Policy and Research (AHCPR publ 91–107), 1991.
24. McGuire LB. A long run for a short jump: understanding clinical guidelines. Ann Intern Med 1990;113:705–708.
25. Health Care Advisory Board. Second generation lessons on critical care paths. Annual meeting, Washington, DC, Dec 1993.
26. CPG strategies: putting guidelines into practice. Chicago: American Hospital Association, Sept 1992.
27. Lomas J, Anderson GM, Dominick-Pierce, et al. Do practice guidelines guide practice. N Engl J Med 1989;321:1306–1311.
28. Kosecoff J, Kanouse DE, Rogers WH, et al. Effects of the National Institutes of Health Consensus Development Program on physicians practice. JAMA 1987;258:2708–2713.
29. Clinton JJ. Improving clinical practice. JAMA 1992;267:2652–2653.
30. Brook RH. Practice guidelines and practicing medicine: are they compatible? JAMA 1989;262:3027–3030.
31. Chassin MR. Standards of care. Inquiry 1988;25:437–453.
32. Eddy DM. Three battles to watch in the 1990's. JAMA 1993;270:520–526.
33. Wennberg JE, Freeman JL, Culp WJ. Are hospitalized services rationed in New Haven or over-utilized in Boston? Lancet 1987;1:1185–1188.
34. Pierce EC. The development of anesthesia guidelines and standards. QRB 1990;16:61–64.
35. Massachusetts Workers' Compensation Law. Massachusetts General Laws, CHAP 152, sec 30, as amended ST. 1991, Chap 398, sec. 53.
36. Smith GH. Maine's Liability Demonstration Project: relating liability to practice parameters. American Medical Association State Health Legislation Report, 1990:1–5.
37. Soumerai SB, Avorn J. Principles of educational outreach to improve clinical decision making. JAMA 1990;263:549–556.
38. The inescapable complexity of decision making: ethics, cost, and informed choices. In: Field MJ, Lolr KN, eds. Guidelines for clinical practice. Washington, DC: National Academy Press, 1992:135–162.

CHAPTER NINE

CLINICAL OUTCOMES

J. Thomas Danzi

It seems that everyone is addressing clinical outcomes as they discuss the need for health care reform. The payers and patients are demanding consistency, accountability, cost containment, and quality in the health care system. Some describe the principal outcome of health care provision as the value of the care. There are six major sponsors of clinical outcomes programs presently. They include health insurance plans, purchasers of health care, health care systems, accrediting organizations, governments, and hospital associations. The challenge is to come to consensus on a definition of clinical outcomes so the data reported are comparable and meaningful. Unfortunately, the present process of data collection without a common definition could cause confusion with the interpretation of the results and possible misrepresentation of the care provided.

The present perception of clinical outcomes resulted from an article written by Paul Ellwood, M.D. and published in the *New England Journal of Medicine* in 1988. The topic of the article was outcomes management, which he defined as "a common patient-understood language of the health outcomes and that estimates the relation between medical intervention and health outcomes as well as the relationship between health outcomes and cost" (1). He described three key activities in the outcome-assessment process: the measurement of indicators; the monitoring of patient characteristics, care processes, and resources related to patient outcome; and management where improved clinical decision making and service delivery relate to optional patient outcomes.

The major impetus for a standardized definition of clinical outcomes has been the requests from patients and payers (insurance companies and HMOs). Today, all purchasers of health care, patients and businesses, want to be able to make an informed decision about what care will be provided and by which physicians. Previously, in the fee-for-service health care market, patients generally decided which practitioner to see on the basis of word-of-mouth reputation, office personnel politeness, and length of wait to be seen. Patient satisfaction is an important outcome of how the care is provided, but it does not correlate with clinical results, patient well-being, or functional status.

The largest group of purchasers of health care—unions, business, and governments—became skeptical of the health care industry's ability to control cost, enhance quality, and provide more consistent care. Their impatience resulted in the emergence of the managed care delivery model in the health care marketplace. Their commitment is acknowledged by the fact that 1993 marked the first time that the number of people covered by traditional indemnity medical insurance was less than 50% of all individuals with employer-sponsored health care (2). This represents almost a 100% increase from 1988, affected by the fact that fewer companies are offering conventional health insurance coverage.

The magnitude of the challenge to define clinical outcome results from the many variables involved in determining the end results of health care provision. Some of the dimensions of clinical outcomes include the efficiency (cost), clinical and functional results, patient well-being, and patient satisfaction. All of these aspects must be evaluated with regard to the time of provision of health care. The result may be different if reviewed immediately after the care, within a year, or up to 3 years later. The monitoring must document the importance of each component of the provider team, including the physician and health care organization, and record patient compliance with treatment or prevention protocols. The methodology to allow a consensus-based definition of clinical outcomes is available with today's medical information systems. The synthesis of clinical, financial, and functional results into a national or regional data bank will, one hopes, allow physicians, patients, and payers to make more rational decisions, based upon a better understanding of the effect of health care decisions on the resultant quality of life.

The reality of a national consensus-based definition of clinical outcomes is years away, close to the turn of the 21st century, because of the need for the six major sponsors of clinical-outcomes programs to complete the process, as outlined by Dr. Ellwood. Fortunately for practicing physicians, this presents an opportunity for the physician community to become proactively involved in the outcome-management process. I am hopeful that my colleagues will respond positively to this challenge and develop a strategy for the medical profession to be an integral part of the clinical-outcomes assessment process.

For the physician community to have meaningful participation in this process, they must first understand the relationship between clinical guidelines, pathways, and clinical outcomes. Many health care organizations, hospitals, and clinics, have asked their physician memberships to participate in developing clinical pathways. Their willingness to become involved in this process has varied from total skepticism to enthusiasm. Most practitioners realized that the eventual reality of this pathway development process could change the manner in which they practice medicine. Fortunately, most medical staffs have the pathway development process led by a group of respected peers who have concluded that their participation was a better alternative than having a payer provide a clinical pathway without their input. While accepting this new reality of clinical practice, the realization of the external and internal review of the care provided clouds the process.

Most organizations presently developing clinical pathways have monitoring plans to assess compliance of health care providers, patients, and operational systems within the pathway. This information will be collected as part of the institution's quality improvement process so it is done in an educational manner. The application of pathways will identify opportunities to enhance the processes of care provision, which will directly improve the clinical results. This process usually results in an improvement of cost indicators for the condition or diagnostic related group (DRG) for which the pathway was developed. Typical cost indicators include length of stay and cost per discharge. It is the rare health care organization that is presently developing clinical pathways in the context of clinical guidelines and projected clinical outcomes. Indeed, if the clinical pathway is the agreed-upon process by which specific care is provided, it is important for the team developing the pathway to first agree on what is the present standard of care for the specific disease. A guideline is a statement summarizing the team's understanding of the present diagnostic and therapeutic options for the specific condition. Commonly, this statement is based upon recommendations from national organizations or societies. Thus, a clinical guideline represents an institution's standard of care for a specific condition. This type of review has educational value for the health care providers participating in the process.

The specific goals of the care provided can be divided into the various categories necessary to satisfy the new clinical outcome requirements that payers and patients are requesting. Having members of the health care team participate in goal setting permits the monitoring process to be one that measures compliance with outcome goals rather than one that evaluates individual providers.

This combination that results in the development of a guideline (standard of care)—a projection of the goals or outcomes of the care provided and a pathway that outlines what and when the care is provided—will permit more physician participation in the clinical-outcomes management process. This methodology is more educational, more apt to yield more cost-efficient higher-quality care provision, and more likely to provide data relative to both the short- and long-term outcomes of the care, as well as being more likely to result in the specific data necessary to resolve questions of patient's functional status, well-being, and satisfaction.

The main challenges that the six major sponsors of clinical-outcomes management projects face are the finalization of the categories of outcomes to be measured and the acceptance of the data collection tools. This may seem easy enough to the novice involved with clinical outcomes, but the success of the project may depend upon the resolution of these two important issues. Before discussing the current status of both of these topics, I shall review some of the legal and ethical issues that must to be resolved before there can be meaningful application of the clinical outcomes data.

One important question involves the confidentiality of the information. Everyone agrees that data must be reported so that no patient can be identified. The debate still continues regarding whether individual practitioners should be compared with their peers or be included in aggregated data of the institution. I believe that since health care teams develop the guideline and pathway and project the goals of care provided, comparisons should be by team rather than by individual. This debate will continue, and whether individual or aggregate data are reported will center on whether the payers and purchasers believe that the medical staff's quality improvement activities can identify and educate physicians who vary from the performance norm of their colleagues.

Another important aspect of outcomes data relates to its discoverability by a court of law. Medical care will improve when its provision closely approximates what the patient desires and what complies with the payer's plan. Since the processes by which care is provided are reviewed within the guidelines of quality improvement, the data should be protected by the Health Care Quality Improvement Act of 1986. Without protection of the information from discoverability, it is my opinion that the true value of the clinical-outcomes management process will not be realized. With its incorporation into the quality improvement process, it is exciting to dream of the meaningful data that could finally be available on clinical outcomes.

The last issue relating to the confidentiality of the data involves the potential input of patient-specific data. It is of concern that patient compliance records could become common knowledge to payers and providers of health care. But if certain individuals have less than desired clinical outcomes because they fail to adhere to specified treatment or wellness protocols, why should the providers (if individual practitioner data are reported) not have the right to know about patient noncompliance if it could affect the provider's report. Many sensitive issues must be resolved regarding the confidentiality of outcomes data.

What is the status of the outcome-measurement projects of the six leading sponsors? All the programs are in the early stages—the definition of the indicators to be measured and preliminary reporting of the measurement. The range of indicators being monitored varies considerably among the initiatives, but there appear to be five general categories of indicators: long-term clinical outcomes, patient satisfaction, efficiency of care, quality of care, and access to care. The indicators addressing long-term outcomes try to assess short- and long-term functional status, patient well-being, and condition-specific incidence of morbidity and mortality after provision of care. The patient satisfaction indicators are intended to define overall satisfaction with the health plan and providers as well as the sensitivity and convenience of the care. The cost or efficiency indicators are designed to provide information on length of service, clinical resource utilization, and administrative costs in the context of the severity of illness. The quality of care or clinical results indicators tend to focus on short-term outcomes (unplanned readmission rates and complication rates), frequency of procedure performance (coronary artery bypass graft, lap cholecystectomy), and compliance with clinical pathways. The indicators designed to assess access to care evaluate the application of prevention and wellness services as well as the waiting time for an office appointment or emergency room visit.

Review of the specific indicators presently being used by the six different types of sponsoring organizations of outcomes management lends insight into their different approaches. The indicators of the Joint Commission on Accreditation of Healthcare Organizations (JCAHO) represent specialty-specific monitors (obstetrics, anesthesia, oncology, cardiovascular, and trauma) or care-specific monitors (medication use, infusion therapy, and infection control). The goal is to allow comparison of hospital-specific data with national and regional standards, and the JCAHO advocates interpreting the data in the context of a quality improvement process. The indicators presently used by hospital associations such as the Maryland Hospital Association assess both inpatient and ambulatory care. Use of the data in a CQI process within hospitals is encouraged.

The indicator systems presently used by health care systems such as Kaiser Permanente and Henry Ford Health System include the National Committee for Quality Assurance's Hedis 2.0 and CRISP indicator assessment process. The orientation of the Hedis 2.0 measuring system is to provide information to employers and consumers to help them decide whether their health plans are meeting their needs, while the objective of the CRISP indictor system is to provide data on a health system's performance. The latter system has indicators that assess population health, community benefit, quality of care, episode prevention, member satisfaction, efficiency, and financial performance. The Hedis 2.0 system provides information on prevention, member health/substance abuse management, patient access and satisfaction, resource utilization, and financial indicators.

It is interesting that health plan sponsors, including health maintenance organizations such as U.S. Healthcare, are tracking indicators similar to those recommended by the Hedis 2.0 system. Most HMOs are seeking data relative to patient access and satisfaction, chronic care management, and preventive services. These organizations have separate informational systems that track clinical resource utilization by providers.

Purchasers of health care can use the previously mentioned outcome measurement systems or develop their own process, as the Cleveland Hospital Quality Council did. In this model, the participating hospital's actual performance is compared with the performance predicted by a statistical model and presented as better, worse, or as expected. This consumer-advocacy project addresses only the inpatient aspect of health care.

Despite the tremendous progress that has been made in clinical outcome measurements, significant concerns still exist. Important questions relate to the accuracy of the data collection and the reliability and validity of the data. Currently, the information is not comparable because it is not adjusted to appropriately reflect differences in patient age, sex, severity of illness, and socioeconomic status. Indeed, conclusions reached with this type of data could undermine the intent of the entire outcomes-management process.

The many questions that currently exist about the collected outcome data show an obvious need for cooperation by the providers and payers of health care in arriving at a consensus definition of a core set of indicators. To date, this collaborative participation in outcomes measurement has been less than ideal. Unfortunately, it may take a legislatively created external authority to mandate and coordinate the process to have standardized definitions.

The cost associated with the data collection for outcomes measurement is important at a time when all administrative costs of health care are being carefully evaluated in terms of its clinical significance. This cost varies, depending on which outcomes-indicator program is used, and is more easily borne by health care systems and large HMOs than by individual hospitals. Until there are meaningful, comparable data, this expense could be interpreted as an unjustified expense.

With the present change in health care thinking to include health, functional status, and patient well-being, the challenge has been to develop accurate health status assessment tools or measures that appropriately reflect the patient's current health and response to health care interventions. This fundamental paradigm shift from disease to health-related assessment is paramount to the success of the clinical-outcomes management process. What assessment tools reflect the physical, mental, and social functioning of the individual as well as his or her perceived well-being? The U.S. Department of Health and Human Service's Healthy People 2000 public policy reflects society's acceptance of health to include an individual's functional capacity and well-being (3). The challenge to health service researchers is to develop new assessment questionnaires that accurately reflect the health of an individual.

A review of past and present health assessment tools reveals that the measures used in the 1960s were predominantly designed to assess only one dimension of health. Assessment centered on either physical or mental health status or was problem/condition specific. There were physical function and disability assessment scales, depression evaluating tools, and classification scales for arthritis (developed by the American Rheumatism Association) and heart disease (developed by New York Heart Association) (4, 5). The development process continued with assessment tools that were easier to complete and began to evaluate the multiple dimensions of health for the first time (6). The most recent tools, developed in the late 1980s, reflect the need for the evaluation process to be brief yet reliable and use a patient questionnaire to assess clinical outcomes (7, 8).

Reporting of the assessment of health status as it relates to clinical practice is beginning. The Agency for Health Care Policy and Research and the Health Outcomes Institute have reported, and will continue to assess, health care provision by the current definition, which includes health status assessment (9, 10).

Currently, many purchasers, payers, and providers of health care are using the SF-36 health status questionnaire. Developed by the RAND Corporation and completed by the patient, it assesses overall perception of health; functional status, physical and emotional; and patient well-being, which addresses the patient's energy and absence of pain. The results provide a subjective impression of the individual's perceived health. The challenge is to combine these data with condition-specific information that addresses severity of illness and the patient's demographic information. The resultant data should more accurately relate the clinical outcome to specific clinical interventions.

One new consideration in the analysis of clinical outcomes is the fact that the health care industry is in an era of mergermania (11). The changes occurring in the latter part of this century indicate that health care in the 21st century will be delivered mainly by large health care systems rather than by individual practitioners or hospitals. The reality of this situation is being driven by the for-profit consolidation of hospital systems at a time when this country appears to have too many inpatient beds. The survivors of this process will probably be systems that have large physician group practices and home care and extended care facilities to offer the entire spectrum of the continuum of care. This tendency to form large health care systems will affect the outcomes-management process currently under way in this country.

A health care system must assess its ability to treat disease and manage health for the full spectrum of care it provides. The challenge is in moving beyond assessing outcomes for each component of the system and tracking across the continuum of care for individuals of all ages.

It should be obvious that there will be no quick solutions to many variables affecting the success of the clinical outcomes management projects. Indeed, the cry for legislative health care reform could potentially impair the process. The payers and purchasers, especially governments, want meaningful clinical-outcomes data today to control the raising cost of health care. The outcomes-management process currently available cannot provide accurate, reliable, meaningful data to achieve this goal. Without common definitions (indicators) or data-collection processes that accurately reflect the severity of illness and the socioeconomic status of the patient, the application of data for this purpose could drastically limit the success of the clinical-outcome review process (12).

Dr. John Wennberg's commentary in 1988 addressed the support required for an effective medical science evaluative process and the time required for appropriate assessment of the outcomes of medical care (13). The leaders of health care reform must ensure that the proper processes are in place to provide outcomes data that can effect the necessary changes in the health care delivery system. The accountability of the health care delivery system in this country must be based on accurate information derived from a uniform assessment process in which the data are stored in a central repository for comparisons (14).

In summary, much progress has been made in the outcomes-management process, but there are still considerable challenges. Unfortunately, assessment of clinical outcomes will require time to confirm the measured data. I am hopeful that my physician colleagues will play an active role in the process and that the proponents of health care reform will give the process of outcomes management the time and resources necessary for its success.

REFERENCES

1. Ellwood P. Shattuck lecture—outcomes management. N Engl J Med 1988;318:1549–1556.
2. Iglehart JK. Health policy report: physicians and the growth of managed care. N Engl J Med 1994;331:1167–1171.
3. U.S. Department of Health and Human Services. Healthy people 2000. DHHS publ (PHS) 91–50213. Washington, DC: U.S. Government Printing Office, 1991.

4. Sternsrocker O, Traeffer CH, Baterman RC. Therapeutic criteria in rheumatoid arthritis. JAMA 1949;140:659.

5. The Criteria Committee of the New York Heart Association. Disease of the heart and blood vessels: nomenclature and criteria for diagnosis. 6th ed. Boston: Little, Brown & Co, 1964.

6. Goldberg DP, Hillier VF. A scaled version of the general health questionnaire. Psychol Med 1979;9:139.

7. Nelson EC, Wasson JH, Kirk JW. Assessment of function in routine clinical practice description of the COOP chart method and preliminary findings. J Chronic Dis 1987; 40(suppl):55S.

8. Stewart AH, Hays RD, Warre JE. The LOS Short-form General Health Survey: reliability and validity in a patient population. Med Care 1988;26:724.

9. Tarlov AR, Ware JE, Greenfield S, et al. The Medical Outcomes Study: an application of methods for monitoring the results of medical care. JAMA 1989;262:295.

10. Research Activities US AHHS, Public Health Service, Agency for Health Care Policy and Research 1990:132.

11. Johnson J. Mega-mergers of hospital. Am Med News 9 Nov 1994:1,35.

12. Oberman L. Reform race spurs scramble for comparison. Am Med News 22 Feb 1993: 3,64,66.

13. Wennberg JE. Improving the medical decision making process. Health Affairs 1988;7:99–106.

14. Ellwood P. The future: clinical outcomes management. In: Couch, JB, ed. Health care quality management in the 21st century. American College of Physician Executive 1994:465–483.

CHAPTER TEN

QUALITY IMPROVEMENT

Neil Schlackman

In spite of the many significant advances in technology and pharmaceuticals in the late 20th century, it is likely that this time period will be remembered for the rapid, evolutionary changes in the health care delivery system—most notably, the extremely swift movement toward managed care. It appears evident that managed care will dominate the delivery of health care well into the 21st century. The structure and processes of managed care will distinguish health care delivery in the United States from that in all other countries. As a response to the significant challenge of moderating costs while greatly expanding access, managed care's approach will be unique among the nations of the world.

Implicit in its name, managed care requires a diffusion of management where previously management has not been a significant aspect of operations. In his health care policy report in 1992 (1), John Iglehart appropriately suggests to physicians that "before doctors reject managed care as too interventionist, they should consider the probable alternatives. In the future, they are likely to face a choice between centralized government regulatory mechanisms, including global budgets, and/or individual incentives for cost control that operate in a pluralistic, privately dominated system. The status quo is not a viable option." Choosing between the two alternative strategies of either regulation (e.g., the government, an all-payer system) or provider and consumer self-control based on incentives (i.e., measuring performance and providing incentives for superior performance) will require an in-depth understanding of the deficits and benefits of each. Those elements of management that potentially threaten the autonomy, prerogative, and authority of the physician can, if appropriately handled, become the instruments of provider self-control as the "managee" becomes the manager. The physician must take initiative to master the myriad new issues involved in "managing" care and create a practice environment in which it is possible not only to survive, but to thrive. The issue for physicians in the 1990s and beyond is to manage or be managed. Accepting this as reality (and not all in medical care have done so in late 1995), physicians must rapidly meet these new challenges effectively to be successful.

The managed care environment has an impact on the clinical side of care in a multitude of ways. An altered philosophy of care and management style is necessary to integrate one's practice into this new milieu. A prominent area of activity in managed care involves the quality assurance (QA)/assessment/improvement process. This chapter attempts to discuss these issues as they affect clinical practice. My approach attempts to meld the demands of the impact of quality improvement activities with the basic framework of clinical practice to improve the delivery of care and describe opportunities for positioning practices for success in this new environment.

Several basic premises underlie the issues facing the American health care system today:

- The more physicians have done, the more they have been paid; thus, there has been an incentive to do more.
- There has been little, if any, incentive for preventive care and little emphasis on quality of care, which is the most productive area of health care.
- No society has the resources to provide all the health services its population is capable of utilizing, yet our society seems to refuse to deal with this critical issue.
- There is an obvious maldistribution of resources, and a large proportion of our population is either uninsured or underinsured.
- Physicians are being asked to practice in a cost-effective manner, adhering to the highest quality standards, in the absence of a "rule book" of how to do so.

The mechanism of payment in prepaid care systems has raised some questions about its effect on the quality of care. A large body of skeptics continue to argue that the quality of care and service in the traditional fee-for-service system is significantly better than that obtained in managed care. The results of considerable health services research paint a different picture. This body of literature (2, 3, 5, 7, 11–13) attempts to evaluate the effect of different payment mechanisms on quality of care. In the fee-for-service system, 20–40% of procedures performed may not be warranted, either because they do not improve health status or because they produce so little improvement that they are not worth the risks or cost (4, 5). Multiple studies (2, 5, 7, 12, 13) comparing fee-for-service and prepaid systems have shown lower use of hospital services in prepaid settings but no consistent differences in either the use of ambulatory services or in the quality of care. Most of these studies were done in "pure" prepaid settings of staff model HMOs (health maintenance organizations) and not in the predominant mode of managed care, the independent practice association model HMO. Independent practice associations (IPAs) and network HMOs presently enroll more than 60% of the more than 50 million HMO members. In two recent studies in which the HMO models were either network or IPA, the quality and quantity of ambulatory care was equal to or better than that for the fee-for-service patients (6, 7). Prepaid care had more colon cancer screening, more annual breast examinations, more biannual mammography, more Papanicolaou smears, better control of hypertension, and better care for congestive heart failure. Researchers at the New England Medical Center and the RAND Corporation have recently published a report of the Medical Outcomes Study which documents that medical specialists who are paid on a fee-for-service basis hospitalize patients more and practice far more expensive medicine than physicians in HMOs (8). It also documented that specialists spent more than family physicians, even when the data are adjusted for severity of illness (9). The structure and the quality improvement activities of the managed care organization appear to enable physicians to improve the quality of care delivered and be far more cost-effective, creating superior value.

Value is what is driving the purchasers of health care today. More and more are convinced that managed care will give them greater value for their health care dollar. They understand that value equals cost and quality. They are deeply disturbed by the questions raised by health care researchers about the consistency and reliability of health services, and they are demanding explicit information about the value of what they are buying. The more sophisticated purchasers such as Xerox, GE, and AT&T are investigating quality before making their purchasing decisions. Health plans, in turn, are demanding that participating practitioners demonstrate their quality. Health plan practitioners are now being held accountable for the quality and quantity of their services in much the same way any other industry is expected to meet the performance specifications of its customers. Those practices that can adapt and provide evidence that they are among the best, as they purport to be, will be the most successful in this brave new world.

The content and focus of traditional QA has changed markedly since the early 20th century. In 1912, Cabot demonstrated the assessment of diagnostic outcomes on the basis of autopsy results. In 1914, Codman demonstrated the assessment of therapeutic outcomes by means of patient follow-up interviews. Over the next 50 years, the structural QA mechanisms of licensure, certification, and accreditation flourished. During the next 25 years, medical chart review methods flourished. This led to a massive regulatory structure that absorbed most of the nation's quality management resources. Avedis Donabedian's landmark conceptualization of health care structure, process, and outcomes is the basis of QA and accepted by most QA professionals. Traditional QA focused on endline inspection using externalized, negative incentives has been met with an atmosphere of fear and defense (10). Inspection-oriented quality programs lead to efforts to discredit rather than learn from the data and to activities that prevent the measurers from uncovering defects in the future. This has resulted in little significant evidence of improvement and tends to subvert the professionalism of quality management.

Distaste for this "bad apple" approach (11) to physician performance has led to the interest in the industrial models emanating from Deming's and Juran's popularization of continuous quality improvement (CQI) or the total quality management (TQM) approach. TQM uses management strategies and scientific methods designed to prevent problems during the production process rather than measuring them after they occur. TQM provides a fundamentally different perspective on the relationship of cost and quality. Until most recently, physicians viewed cost as irrelevant in their decision making. Medical education fostered the belief that increased quality required increased cost. In a variety of industries, TQM has proven that true improvements in quality lead to lower cost. The scientific methods of TQM are built on the premise that reducing inappropriate variation and complexity will result in higher quality and lower cost.

The problem-solving approach with which most health care providers are becoming familiar involves

- Identifying priorities or hypotheses to test
- Testing the hypotheses to confirm a correctable problem or improvement plan
- Identifying factors essential for improvement plan
- Implementing the plan
- Reevaluating to determine the impact

As the health care system has become more monitored and scrutinized by payers, purchasers, and patients, practitioners find themselves increasingly compared with each other. When faring poorly, they plead: "My patients are sicker, and I provide the best care, so I attract the sicker patients." This defense has placed a significant impediment in the path of those who question practitioners' performance. Even in the 1910s, Codman acknowledged the importance of adjusting for patient risk, and since that time, an entire industry has emerged to measure "severity of illness." The goal of this "risk adjustment" is to control for the confounding influence of patient severity in comparisons of outcomes that might be related to severity. There are a variety of systems available, but no consensus on a single definition of severity exists. This lack of consensus reflects the realities and the uncertainties of current medical practice and knowledge. This entire concept is new to most physicians and needs to be understood and incorporated into present day practice to be successful in the new world of managed care.

There are over 550 HMOs and countless PPOs and other arrangements in the medical marketplace today. This presents a confusing array of choices for the consumer, the employer, and the physician. With competition increasing among health care plans, employees of large firms are typically faced with more choices and more complex options than in the past. There is a perception in the medical marketplace that consumers make rational choices among alternatives. Unfortunately, other than cost and coverage information, there is a paucity of clear information on any other dimension. Some important influences on choice appear to be the physician/patient relationship, the cost of the plan (often without information about cost-sharing data and out-of-pocket costs), and other perceived individual or family needs. Purchasers want reliable and comparable information, beginning with process measures, but moving on to outcomes. They want evidence that the plan uses its findings to improve quality. Thus, quality must be defined in a some more objective fashion. The recent efforts by the National Committee for Quality Assurance (NCQA) (12) in spearheading the development of accreditation of health plans and also, as a distinct effort, performance measures, represented by the Health Plan Employer Data and Information Set (HEDIS) (13) have added an important resource for purchasers.

NCQA is a nonprofit organization that represents a unique partnership of health plans, consumers, purchasers and health services researchers. The NCQA accreditation process will have evaluated approximately one-half of the 550 HMOs in the United States by the beginning of 1996. This extensive on-site evaluation reviews six distinct areas within the health plan: quality improvement, credentialing, utilization review, members' rights and responsibilities, medical records, and preventive health. The ultimate goal is to evaluate the internal quality processes of the health plan with regard to its ability to improve the quality of health care delivery in that plan. Many purchasers are beginning to require NCQA accreditation as a prerequisite for being offered to a purchaser's employees. The fact that the standards for these areas are valued much more toward the optimal end of the spectrum than when minimal or average has created a dramatic need for health plans to request and require practices/providers to adhere to high standards that are much more explicit than they have been accustomed to in their relatively insulated practice environments. In fact, only about 30% of reviewed plans have received full accreditation in mid-1995. The most significant of the standards is in the area of quality improvement. It requires the plan to provide evidence of effectiveness of its programs. Since participating physician practices are the nidus for the demonstration of effectiveness, those practices that understand the elements of the quality improvement process and can demonstrate clear evidence of superior performance will be the most valued. They will win in an arena where there will be clear winners and losers. After all, part of the definition of managed care includes the aspects of the free enterprise system or capitalism, where there always are winners and losers. Medical care is finally coming into the 20th century as far as economic reality, even as the rest of the economy approaches the 21st century.

HEDIS was initiated by the purchaser community in 1989. It should be differentiated from the accreditation process, for it attempts to assess performance of a health plan according to a specified set of measures. Although there are over 60 different measures, including clinical quality and access, patient satisfaction, membership and finance, and utilization, the quality measures have the greatest impact on the practicing physician. The areas of quality evaluated are preventive services (e.g., immunizations, Papanicolaou testing, mammography, prenatal care, acute and chronic care (e.g., asthma admission rate, diabetic retinal examination rate), and mental health. HEDIS is an excellent beginning even though it uses primarily process measures rather than outcome measures. As HEDIS develops—it is in its infancy now with many limitations—it will become more useful and enhance the ability of purchasers and consumers to choose a health plan. Because the HEDIS data set is drawn from the practices that participate with the plan, practitioners who actively participate in this quality improvement process will be the most valued and successful.

The ultimate consumer of health care, the patient, should not be forgotten. The fact that consumers often choose a health plan for reasons other than the primary physician may create difficulties in establishing a positive physician-patient relationship. Choosing a practitioner's name out of a book presents a different set of preferences than a recommendation from a present patient or another physician. Physicians must learn to adapt to this method of physician selection and develop mechanisms to enhance the physician/patient relationship that they may not have used in the past. Introductory letters, office brochures, open houses, etc. are more necessary than ever before. An introductory or "get acquainted" visit extolling the virtues of the practice and describing the major aspects of the specific plan the patient is covered by is a new experience for most physicians, but a critical one in this day and age.

Over 90% of HMOs use primary care physicians as gatekeepers (14). The term *gatekeeper* has been viewed in pejorative terms and has implied the bureaucratic function of limiting high-cost medical services. Approximately 75% of medical services appear to be managed by primary care physicians (15). Gatekeeping should be viewed as the "matching of patients' needs and preferences with the judicious use of medical services" (16). The primary care physician guides the patient through the complex health care system. This suggests that the gatekeeper makes decisions about appropriate and necessary care and protects the patient from the adverse effects of unnecessary and inappropriate care. In part, the risks of care have risen as a result of the increasing intensity of the care provided. This has been due to several interrelated factors. Fee-for-service medicine operates under the premise that "the more you do, the more you are paid." Technical skills are rewarded more than are cognitive skills. The increase in malpractice litigation has increased the apparent need for more intensive care. New technology is often added to the old technology and is often adopted without evidence that it improves outcomes. Professional uncertainty about the "right" decision often leads to the pursuit of diagnostic certainty beyond clinical usefulness. There is an oversupply of specialists who set the standards by their diagnostic and procedure-oriented approach.

Physicians in HMOs provide less intense care in both ambulatory (17) and hospital setting (18) than is provided by fee-for-service physicians. Primary care physicians provide less intense care for similar severity-of-illness patients than specialists, with no difference in outcomes (5). Not only are HMO patients less likely to be hospitalized, but the HMOs provide a quality of care that is equal or superior to that in the fee-for-service setting (3). Although the "perverse incentive" (i.e., limiting resources when income is linked to limitation of resource use) has been greatly publicized, there is little evidence that primary care physicians withhold beneficial care for financial reasons. There is evidence to support the thesis that primary care physicians are more likely to provide continuity and comprehensiveness of care than are specialists. Data also indicate that primary care physicians are more likely to identify patients who are not appropriate candidates for a procedure more effectively than specialists who perform the procedure (7). Thus, it is reasonable to conclude that gatekeeping by primary care physicians is a critical part of an optimally functioning health care system.

Many managed care plans consider gatekeeper requirements to be a major source of managed care efficiency. The days of American physicians practicing medicine unfettered by concerns of cost are rapidly vanishing. The medical profession's traditional resistance to setting limits in any form is unlikely to remain a credible position (19). Physician involvement in selecting cost-containment strategies that best preserve professional integrity and minimize disruption of patient care will be far more productive. It has been argued that physicians in "gatekeeper systems" serve a "rationing" function that may lead to an adversarial doctor-patient relationship. Traditional fee-for-service medicine requires no input from the primary physician for appropriate referral, which may lead to unnecessary care and increased iatrogenic disease. Patients who want or need direct access to specialized care are less likely to tolerate the gatekeeper role of making referrals. Occasionally, physicians may steer "costly" patients away from gatekeeper programs that frustrate such patients' direct access to specialized care. Many medical practices have not been accustomed to carrying out the case management role envisioned for gatekeepers.

Physicians frequently wave the banner of professional autonomy with great flourish and lack of precision. The era of absolute "clinical freedom," which is the ability of the physician to deliver medical care to a patient without the uninvited imposition of outside influences, is over. Quality assurance/assessment/improvement activities, whose goals are the improvement of patient care, should not be construed as a loss of autonomy. The gatekeeper can open the "gate" to appropriate referrals or close it to inappropriate ones. Theoretically, the primary physician is fully aware of all care a patient receives. However, physicians in traditional fee-for-service medicine have limited knowledge of the sources of care their patients obtain. The opportunity for patients to self-refer often creates great fragmentation of care and little opportunity for medically directed decision making regarding the appropriateness or the need for the resource selected. Although there is the potential for disagreement with the patient about the necessity or desire for referral to specialist or hospital services, the primary physician as a gatekeeper in managed care is much more aware of the need for and the direction of the medical care of his or her patients.

The relationship of primary physicians and specialists may change dramatically in managed care. The proliferation of primary care gatekeeper arrangements can create a tension between primary physicians and referral specialists. Specialists are concerned about the ability of primary care physicians to perform some of the care they feel should be relegated only to them. At the same time, primary physicians express concern about the referral specialists' lack of recognition of the broader needs of the patient. A major deficit in our traditional health care system is the fragmentation of care that often occurs when specialists manage care with minimal or no communication to the primary physician. Similarly, the primary physician needs to communicate patients' needs and concerns to the specialist to achieve the optimal outcome for patients. Since managed care requires the direct involvement of the primary physician in the referral process, this necessitates closer communication between the primary and specialist physician, as well as with the patient. Professional collegiality is at risk in the highly competitive market for medical care. Tensions between primary physicians and specialists increase as many primary physicians involved in gatekeeper and capitation arrangements redistribute income and power. For primary physicians, this moves them back toward the central position in the delivery system. For specialists, it creates an environment requiring increased communication and the recognition of increased competition. Ultimately, this should enhance the quality of care and services, improve patient outcomes and lower costs.

Today there are two markedly different regulatory approaches to cost containment: expenditure targets (global budgetary controls) and utilization review. Utilization review provides a negative incentive for providing certain services (e.g., noncoverage or nonpayment). A major deficit in this process is the uncertainty about what constitutes appropriate care. Several studies have confirmed this lack of agreement (20, 21). In the RAND studies of appropriateness of certain procedures, there was significant disagreement among the experts about appropriateness (22). Moreover, it is daunting to think that one will be able to review over 350 million claims from 500,000 physicians for over 7,000 different procedure codes with any consistency. Thus, utilization review of every episode of care is neither reasonable nor feasible.

Strict utilization review linked to payment decisions is a singularly American approach to cost control; expenditure targets or caps are prominent cost-containment strategies in Canada and Germany. This alternative to utilization review is a global boundary that sets clear limits on the amount of money budgeted for the health system. International experience suggests that this is much more effective because it avoids the bureaucracy required by utilization review. Global limits focus on the collective behavior of large groups of physicians and patients, rather than on individual physician/patient encounters. While global limits delineate boundaries that circumscribe the ultimate clinical freedom "to do everything possible," these boundaries distance the cost-control process from day-to-day clinical decisions. Global budgetary methods allow physicians to exercise internal professional review, perhaps using medical practice parameters, against a few outliers, while utilization review requires outside agents to scrutinize the daily decisions of all physicians. This is not to imply that global budgets are necessarily effective in controlling costs.

An additional approach is to utilize many of the elements that have been said to define quality, measure them and reward them. Using these measurements to provide an incentive to practitioners may be another mechanism to avoid limitation on clinical freedom (23, 24). No cost-containment approach will be entirely free of erosion of clinical autonomy. However, it would appear that global budgeting and creating incentives for optimal behavior represent more effective and less intrusive alternatives.

Many physicians have considered managed care contracting as an obstacle to clinical and financial autonomy. Selective physician contracting, as practiced in many managed care organizations, has provoked physicians' complaints of exclusion from managed care plans and led to the support of legislation that would severely restrict the ability of certain managed care organizations to contract preferentially or use gatekeeper programs. The addition of certain credentialing policies to distinguish among eligible physicians has caused anxiety in the medical community. On the other hand, many physician groups have begun to assume greater risk for both the cost and quality of care, and it will be interesting to observe their reaction to the legislation that they supported, as they may be required to accept "any willing provider." While physicians may feel pressured by economic necessity to participate in managed care, relatively few philosophically support the underlying premise of a competitive market; fewer still are prepared or knowledgeable enough to take "reasoned risks." Physicians' reaction to the intrusion of managed care bears a striking resemblance to the grieving process identified by Kubler-Ross in the transition from denial to anger to depression to bargaining and acceptance. Nonetheless, to succeed in the last decade of the 90s, physicians must understand the mechanics of compensation systems and performance evaluations and become actively involved in the decisions related to their development and implementation.

Underlying the measurement of performance, which may drive the choice of physicians in a plan and the potential rewards received, is a concept of focusing on the patterns of care provided by physicians rather than individual occurrences of care. The concept of focusing on patterns of care has been labeled "physician profiling" (25). Profiling has emerged as an important mechanism in these diverse efforts. Information obtained from large databases is used to identify a provider's pattern of practice and compare it with patterns of similar providers or with an accepted standard or benchmark. The practice pattern of a single physician or a group is expressed as a rate: some measure of the use of resources during a defined period for the population served (26). The American College of Physicians, in its proposal for universal insurance (27), and Congress (28), in its 1989 Medicare physician-payment reform, have advocated physician profiling. Profiling is viewed as a potentially effective tool to identify excesses and deficiencies in care, to target ways of improving the efficiency and quality of care, and to assess provider performance.

The reasons for the expanding use of profiling include its broad applicability, the growing availability of data on which it can be based, and the spread and improvement of technology for processing this information. The availability of information may be outpacing the ability to use profiling effectively and responsibly. As profiling has become more widespread, diverse groups have raised concerns over the quality of the profiles themselves, the uses to which they have been put, and access to the information contained in them.

Profiling uses epidemiologic methods to compare practice patterns on the dimensions of cost, service use, or quality of care and service. The mechanics of profiling can be applied to an individual practitioner, a group of practitioners, or a health care organization. The number of specific claims submitted per 100 patients a physician sees per year is an example of a profiling rate. Comparisons in profiling are made by relating the utilization or outcome rate for a particular practitioner to a norm, which can be either a rate derived from the practice patterns of other similar practitioners (a practice-based norm) or a rate that would be expected if providers followed an accepted practice guideline (a standard-based norm). Practice-based norms do not necessarily reflect appropriate care. The rate at which practitioners provide a particular service may be too high or too low. Standards-based norms reflect appropriate care to the extent that they are based on practice guidelines grounded in sound scientific evidence.

Profiling should be accompanied by some kind of action that may be taken if the utilization or outcome rate for a particular practitioner differs from the norm by a certain amount. For example, a particular practitioner might be notified if the rate of performing a particular procedure is greater than two standard deviations above the mean for physicians practicing in the same community. If a standard-based norm is available, physicians might be told the extent to which their rates are appropriate or inappropriate (i.e., whether their rates meet the norm or are too high or too low in relation to it). The potential of profiling relates to the way it can theoretically be applied in three important areas: quality improvement, assessment of provider performance, and utilization review.

The goal of quality improvement is to identify problems and overcome them by changes in performance. Problems in health care may be indicated by poor or variable patient outcomes. Methods for improving outcomes may require changes in any or all of the partners in the health care team—the physicians, nonphysician practitioners, hospitals, other institutional providers, patients, and/or health care systems. Profiling can play a role in several aspects of quality improvement. It can be used to target potential problem areas by identifying conditions or procedures in which there are variations in outcome (such a profile would measure differences in the frequency with which a specific outcome occurs when patients with a particular condition or patients undergoing a particular procedure are cared for by different providers). Welch et al. recently showed that large databases can detect differences in practice among individual physicians as well as among groups (29).

It can also be helpful in determining how and by whom performance should be changed to improve outcome. Through feedback of the results of an outcomes profile, practitioners may be able to identify specific differences in the processes of care (not necessarily attributable to them) that are likely to underlie the differences in outcomes. These hypotheses can then be tested by running profiles on both the process and the outcome of care, looking for correlations between the two, and/or modifying the process of care across practitioners to see if on reprofiling differences in outcomes are reduced or overall outcome is improved. Surgeons in Maine have demonstrated that feedback about practice style suffices to bring extreme values into line (30).

Valid methods for assessing provider performance are important to many parties for a wide variety of purposes. They can provide a basis for choosing physicians, hospitals, and health plans (by consumers and payers); making decisions about certification, credentialing, and granting of hospital privileges; monitoring compliance with outcomes of practice guidelines or quality improvement measures; assessing the effectiveness of medical training; and identifying areas that may require more effective undergraduate, graduate, or continuing medical education. Profiling can potentially play an important role in this regard, since it can be used to identify practitioners who do not meet a certain standard of care. For a particular condition or procedure, it may be possible to identify a specific process measure(s) that is associated with appropriate, cost-effective care. A particular practitioner's utilization rate for this service could be compared with the rate that would be expected for practitioners who followed the guideline. Performance would be "acceptable" if the practitioner's rate does not deviate substantially from this norm.

The opportunity to maintain contracts with physicians on the basis of explicit performance data holds more promise and perhaps greater fear for the physician community. The ability to channel large segments of services to specified practitioners on the basis of performance data, theoretically, would improve the efficiency and quality of care. The ability to distinguish among physicians to reward better-performing physicians is a major advantage of managed care organizations and a potential threat to independent physicians who do not participate in those systems. Physicians must be involved in the definitions of optimal performance, which must be based on sound scientific evidence for the "reward" to be valid.

An added task required of the physician in managed care is to integrate information that was not previously considered in the days of "unmanaged" care. The need for exceptional management information systems is evident and usually not available to most practitioners. Provision of administrative data, such as reports on pharmaceutical use by patients, is a potent source of information that may be used to improve quality of care. Provision of peer-comparison feedback on the practice's hospital, specialist, and emergency room utilization is common in managed care. Providing utilization information to enable practices to effectively manage care is a major advance. Most physicians will have to learn to deal with and effectively use this information, which has the potential for better, more cost-effective care.

Historically, the medical profession has focused on disease and its treatment rather than its prevention, and on the pathogenesis of poor health rather than the promotion of good health. Lifestyle and behavior are central to the development of major chronic diseases. The notion of primary prevention is something that most physicians still relegate to the domain of public health. The great challenge for physicians is to pay more attention to helping patients adopt healthy behavior. However, reducing patients' risk factors poses a particular challenge to primary care physicians. To accomplish health promotion and disease prevention in the clinical setting, physicians will have to provide education and counseling for behavior change, anticipatory guidance, screening tests to detect presymptomatic disease, immunizations, and chemoprophylaxis.

The U.S. Preventive Services Task Force *Guide to Clinical Preventive Services* provides a blueprint for the delivery of these services (31). This is the product of over 4-years review, and it evaluates the effectiveness of 169 health promotion and disease prevention interventions. The influence of this guide will be determined by how widely physicians adopt the recommendations and follow them in practice. There are several barriers to implementation:

- Limited communication of these and other guidelines to practicing physicians.
- Physicians have been trained to be problem solvers and focus on the symptomatic patient.

- Physicians and patients tend to discount the value of a future gain when compared with the immediate reward for treatment.
- Traditional reimbursement policies value diagnosis and treatment and neither value nor compensate for health promotion.

Typically, physicians have been skeptical about the objectivity of groups creating recommendations. Managed care organizations' use of well-formulated, appropriately applied guidelines can serve to diminish conflict and increase the confidence of physicians in using them. In traditional independent practice, there is little support available for health promotion. If there is an expanded array of clinical preventive services, it may be perceived as adding work rather than expanding professional roles. Managed care can involve the patient in educational and interventional activities outside the physicians' offices. This may be perceived as an intrusion in the practice of medicine or as an aid to the interventions desired. This educational opportunity may enhance the physician's ability to provide more comprehensive care to the patient (e.g., information about mammography, Papanicolaou testing, breast self-examination, poisoning, smoking cessation). Physicians should adapt to this change in the direction of health care information and learn to utilize the potential support of the managed care organization.

Focused education for the physician is another opportunity that managed care often makes available. Programs such as the counterdetailing utilized by Avorn and Soumerai to produce significant decreases in prescribing habits for overused drugs have been quite effective (32). Feedback about performance, individually and compared with peers, and group performance appears to improve physician compliance with peer-preestablished criteria or "standards of care" (e.g., cesarean section rates, use of pelvimetry) (33, 34). Common elements of these successful interventions are the use of individualized, specific, and timely feedback. Physicians may feel that these programs intrude on their autonomy. With the intent of quality improvement, the managed care organization must develop these programs with physician input and introduce them in a nonthreatening manner. The programs must provide valid, credible, and reproducible material of value to the physician. In an attempt to maximize the effectiveness of these programs, some health plans have begun to provide some form of incentive for superior performance.

A difficult issue has been the reasonable and appropriate role for patient involvement in the medical care process. The challenge is to balance the values of patients and the autonomy of physicians. There are two distinct roles for patients: as evaluators of care and as active participants in care. There is evidence that including patients in their care can positively affect its quality, measured even in clinical terms.

Empirical evidence has shown that patients usually give their physicians high ratings for the care they receive. On a scale of 1 to 100, patients will characteristically give their care scores of 82 or above. However, small differences, even at the top end of the spectrum, have important implications for patients' subsequent behavior with respect to health and health care (e.g., an 8-point difference at the high end of the spectrum was associated with a 10-fold increase in the probability of disenrollment from a health plan (35)). Several studies have shown that although patients' assessments of care tend to be consistently higher than the ratings of that same care by physicians and nurses, care judged as excellent or good by physicians or nurses is also similarly judged by patients. Recent research indicates that patients are rating something real when they value interpersonal care and that better interpersonal care does have clinical relevance. Studies are under way to sort out the relationship of patient's ratings of their health care to their health outcomes. However, there is considerable evidence that patients' assessments of care have important consequences for their health and for the health care they receive. Dissatisfied patients are more likely to engage in behavior that could disrupt their health outcomes (e.g., physician shopping, disenrollment from their health plan, initiating frivolous malpractice claims, self-directed care). There is some limited research to indicate that feedback to practitioners of overall scores from patients' evaluations leads to subsequent improvements in their scores (29).

Although patient participation in care has been very limited and has not had a smooth history, there are several reasons why patient participation is important (36). With respect to access and to the patient-physician relationship, patients' evaluations of the quality of care they receive are the most practical source of information. Over 10 years of empirical research (most importantly by J. Ware) (37) has produced valid and reliable measures of patient satisfaction with medical care that can be used in practice settings. Patients' assessments of care have been shown to affect both the physician-patient relationship and patients' health status. Research has shown a link between clinical measures of health and patient-reported health outcomes (e.g., better control of blood sugar and FEV1 have been associated with better levels of self-reported functioning) (38). There is evidence that patients want an expanded role in their medical care and that this expanded role may produce better outcomes (39–41). Finally, there are several major efforts under way that use patient assessments of care to evaluate the delivery of health care (e.g., American Board of Internal Medicine uses such data for certification, as well as incentive systems in managed health care.) Thus, it is an appropriate time to consider the role of patient satisfaction in the assessment of quality.

For all these reasons, some managed care organizations have turned to the use of patient satisfaction data as one mechanism for rewarding quality care. Patient satisfaction should be considered to be one of the desired outcomes of care. It is futile to argue about the validity of patient satisfaction as a measure of quality. Whatever its strengths and limitations as a measure of quality, information about patient satisfaction should be used as a tool to improve patient care in the areas that patients find important. Physicians will have to learn to use this new information constructively and not allow the threat to their egos to impair the opportunity for improving the care and service they provide.

There is a growing demand for information describing the "correct" medical care, or "guidelines." Multiple groups and agencies are attempting to structure these guidelines. For the last 20 years, studies by Wennberg and colleagues and others have documented large inconsistencies in the rate at which specific procedures are performed in different areas of the country (42, 43). For example, Wennberg found that carotid endarterectomies are performed twice as often in residents of Boston than in residents of New Haven. Conversely, residents of New Haven have twice the rate of coronary bypass operations of their Boston counterparts (44).

The Agency for Health Care Policy and Research (AHCPR) was established by Congress in 1990 as a major effort to convene experts for the creation of guidelines that would help physicians reduce treatment uncertainty, eliminate inappropriate choices, and improve patient outcomes. In 1991, the AHCPR convened 13 expert panels and contracted for three guidelines. In addition to variations based on differences in patients' health status, there are still substantial variations in clinical practice that stem from professional uncertainty, lack of knowledge, differences in training, and individual physician decision making. These variations may contribute to misallocation of resources and available services. These discrepancies have also been cited for putting patients at risk and driving up the cost of care with unnecessary treatment. Health and Human Services Secretary Louis Sullivan described research to develop treatment guidelines as "the beginning of a peaceful revolution in American medical care." Whether it is peaceful and how much of a revolution occurs will depend to a great extent on the manner of implementation of these guidelines and their perceived utility in practice.

Although the American Medical Association supports the guidelines and the federal medical effectiveness effort, it has warned against using the guidelines as "cookbook" medicine. The AHCPR has no regulatory authority to require doctors to follow any of its recommendations, but it is expected that the guidelines will have an effect similar to that of the recommendations of the Centers for Disease Control. There is a possibility that funding for this agency may not survive the late 1990s budget-cutting process. It is quite likely that Medicare and other third-party payers will use the guidelines in making reimbursement decisions. Managed care organizations should be able to apply these guidelines in a uniform fashion as they become more useful and, one hopes, improve the quality of care, protect professional autonomy, reduce litigation risk, minimize practice variation, create credible audits of care, and decrease cost by their use.

Until recently, as the custodian of its own standards, the medical profession has attained a very high degree of autonomy. It has been able to determine its own working conditions and terms of payment and has been successful, until recently, in making medical decisions immune from outside examination. However, as a result of the extraordinary cost of medical care, there is less willingness to accept the word of the medical "expert," especially in face of the documented enormous overuse of inappropriate or unnecessary services and underuse of appropriate ones. Purchasers want accountability for the huge resources used, and in the absence of some means to cap expenditures (e.g., the Canadian budget experience), their only recourse is to review individual decisions of physicians. No longer will they leave judgments concerning quality to the medical profession alone. The heightened awareness and desire for information on quality and the difficulty involved in measuring it have made practitioners and purchasers uncomfortable. Physicians resent this review and do not like to be measured or monitored. Physicians must begin to accept the legitimacy of the concern about the cost and quality of medical care. Managed care can assist physicians to learn and apply the new "rules" and become more effective participants. Interacting with these rules and working toward the goal of objective quality improvement is a bold new task for physicians. Those that accept this challenge will be professionally and financially successful.

In addition to the generic issue of guidelines or clinical effectiveness, there is a new mandate to value what has been called "outcomes management" in the performance of physicians. Paul Ellwood has described outcomes management as a "technology of patient experience designed to help patients, payers, and providers make rational medical-care choices based on better insight into the effect of these choices on the patient's life" (45). Outcomes management uses standards or guidelines, attempts to measure functioning and well-being, pools this information for use as a resource, and analyzes and disseminates the results. In the most optimistic appraisal there is hope that a bridge can be built between the real time data needed by physicians to monitor and improve their daily medical practice and the retrospective data used by insurers to control the cost and quality of covered services. Several managed care organizations have tried to integrate a variety of these measures into their payment mechanism. As Paul Ellwood said, "Only physicians have the full opportunity to use outcomes management as a technology of experience to enhance their own knowledge of the decisiveness of science and the subtlety of caring to bring a better quality of life to their patients." The limitations of outcomes research should not deter plans from pursuing this rational approach to the assessment of medical care (46). These issues have important implications for the relationship between patient and physician as they are integrated into the financing of health care.

The RAND Corporation and the UCLA Department of Medicine have collaborated with the HMO Quality Assessment Consortium, which comprises 11 leading HMOs, and have identified nine aspects of medical care that should be assessed as part of the evaluation of quality: access, use of services, symptoms, interpersonal aspects of care, technical aspects of care, diagnostic tests, medications, patient education, and outcomes of care (40). Utilizing a variety of sources, managed care organizations are beginning to use these data elements to value quality (47). There is an interesting and evolving tension between the traditional arm's-length relationship between a managed care organization and a physician in private practice and the managed care organization's ethical, and increasingly legal, need to evaluate the quality of care provided by that physician.

In 1978 the Institute of Medicine (IOM) highlighted several characteristics it defined as essential components of quality primary care practice: accessibility, comprehensiveness, coordination, continuity, and accountability (48). Although these concepts are difficult to translate into quantifiable scientific measures of doctors' performance, some innovative managed care organizations are beginning to develop such measures. The ability to gather and analyze large quantities of data from a variety of sources—claims data, audits of medical care, pharmacy information, laboratory data, patient-satisfaction surveys—will allow possible ratings of individual physicians over time. The goal should be the continuous improvement of care and service. The benefit extends to the patient, the doctor, the employer, and the managed care organization.

Competitive health care delivery demands valid and reliable quality of care measures that can be used to compare health plans. For comparisons to be fair and useful for purchasers and policy makers, it makes sense to use measures of quality that are population-based, independent of practice style or setting of care, and balanced with respect to assessing under- or overprovision of services. The availability and use of such measures would help consumers and major purchasers compare health care organizations on the basis of quality issues in addition to cost. Indeed, the public availability of comparative quality of care data could provide an incentive for plans and physicians to adopt quality management or "continuous improvement" strategies designed to enhance performance. We might heed

Benjamin Franklin, who in 1776 told his colleagues, "If we do not hang together, we most assuredly will hang separately."

Managed care is a viable solution to the health care crisis, and physicians who use its tools can become the appropriate managers of their own destinies. Physicians need to understand and to be involved in this process, or as Yogi Berra is quoted as saying, "If you don't know where you are going, you could end up somewhere else."

ACKNOWLEDGMENTS

Selected portions of Schlackman N. The impact of managed care on clinical practice. In: Bloomberg MA, Mohlie SR, eds. Physicians in managed care. Tampa: American College of Physician Executives, were used in this chapter with permission.

The views and opinions expressed herein are those of Dr. Schlackman and do not necessarily reflect the views, opinions and policies of U.S. Healthcare, Inc.

REFERENCES

1. Iglehart JK. Health policy report: the American health care system: managed Care. N Engl J Med. 1992:327:742–747.
2. Hillman AL, Pauly MV, Kerman K, Martinek CR. HMO managers' views on financial incentives and quality. Health Aff 1991:10(4):207–219.
3. Sui AL, Sonnenberg FA, Manning WG, Goldberg GA, Bloomfield ES. Inappropriate use of hospitals in a randomized of health insurance plans. N Engl J Med 1986;315:1259–1266.
4. Chassin MR, Kosecoff J, Park RE, et al. Does inappropriate use explain geographic variations in the use of health services? A study of three procedures. JAMA 1987;258:2533–2537.
5. Kosecoff J, Chassim MR, Fink A, et al. Obtaining clinical data on the appropriateness of medical care in community practice. JAMA 1987;258:2538–2542.
6. Udvarhelyi IS, Jennison K, Phillips RS, Epstein AM. Comparison of the quality of ambulatory care for fee-for-service and prepaid patients. Ann Intern Med 1991;115:394–400.
7. Retchin SM, Brown B. Elderly patients with congestive heart failure under prepaid care. Am J Med 1991;90:236–242.
8. Greenfield S, Nelson EC, Zubkoff M, et al. Variations in resource utilization among medical specialties and systems of care. Results from the medical outcomes study. JAMA 1992;267:1624–1630.
9. Kravitz RL, Greenfield S, Rogers W, et al. Differences in the mix of patients among medical specialties and systems of care. Results from the medical outcomes study. JAMA 1992;267:1617–1623.
10. Berwick DM, Wald DL. Hospital leaders' opinions of the HCFA mortality data. JAMA 1990;263:247–249.
11. Berwick DM. Continuous improvement as an ideal in health care. N Engl J Med 1989; 320:53–6.
12. National Committee for Quality Assurance. NCQA reviewer guidelines, standards for accreditation, 1995. 2000 L Street, NW, Suite 500, Washington, DC 20036.
13. National Committee for Quality Assurance. Health plan employer data and information set and users' manual, version 2.0, 1993. 2000 L Street, NW, Suite 500, Washington, DC 20036.
14. Langwell KM. Structure and performance of health maintenance organizations: a review. Health Care Financ Rev 1990;12(1):71–79.

15. Deitrich AJ, Nelson EC, Kirk JW, Zubkoff M, O'Connor GT. Do primary physicians actually manage their patients' fee-for-service care? JAMA 1988;259:3145–3149.
16. Franks P, Clancy CM, Nutting PA. Gatekeeping revisited—protecting patients from over-treatment. N Engl J Med 1992;327:424–429.
17. Epstein AM, Begg CB, McNeil BJ. The use of ambulatory testing in prepaid and fee-for-service group practices. Relation to perceived profitability. N Engl J Med 1986;314: 1089–1094.
18. Johnson AN, Dowd B, Morris NE, Lurie N. Differences in inpatient resource use by type of health plan. Inquiry 1989;26:388–98.
19. Stych E. After years of combat AMA accepts HMOs. (Associated Press) Philadelphia Inquirer. Friday, June 12, 1992.
20. Dippe SE, Bell MM, Wells MA, Lyons W, Clester S. A peer review of a peer review organization. West J Med 1989;151:93–96.
21. Goldman RL. The reliability of peer assessments of quality of care JAMA 1992;267: 958–960.
22. Park RE, Fink A, Brook RH, et al. Physician ratings of appropriate indications for three procedures: theoretical indications vs indications used in practice. Am J Public Health 1989;79:445–447.
23. Schlackman N. Integrating quality assessment and physician incentive payment. QRB 1989;5:234–237.
24. Schlackman N. Evolution of quality-based compensation model—the third generation. Am J Med Quality. Summer 1993;8:103–110.
25. Lasker RD, Shapiro DW, Tucker AM. Realizing the potential of practice pattern profiling. Inquiry 1992;24:287–297.
26. Lee PR, Shapiro DW, Lasker RD, Bindman AB. Managed care provider profiling. J Insur Med 1992;24:179–181.
27. Scott HD, Shapiro HB. Universal insurance for American health care: a proposal of the American College of Physicians. Ann Intern Med 1992;117:511–519.
28. Omnibus Budget Reconciliation Act of 1989, 42 U.S.C. 1395u(b)(3)(L).
29. Welch HG, Miller ME, Welch WP. Physician profiling: an analysis of inpatient practice patterns in Florida and Oregon. N Engl J Med 1994;330:607–612.
30. Keller RB, Chapin AM, Soule DN. Informed inquiry into practice variations: the Maine Medical Assessment Foundation. Qual Assur Health Care 1990;2:69–75.
31. U.S. Preventive Services Task Force, Guide to clinical preventive services: an assessment of the effectiveness of 169 interventions. Baltimore: Williams & Wilkins, 1989.
32. Avorn J, Soumerai SB. Improving drug-therapy decision through educational outreach. N Engl J Med 1983;308:1457–1463.
33. Chassin MR, McCue SM. A randomized trial of medical quality assurance. Improving physician's use of pelvimitry. JAMA 1986;256:1012–1016.
34. Stafford RS. Alternative strategies for controlling rising cesarean section rates. JAMA 1990;263:683–687.
35. Ware JE Jr, Davies AR. Behavioral consequences of patient dissatisfaction with medical care. Eval Prog Planning 1983;6:291–297.
36. Nash DB, Goldfield N, eds. The patient's role in health care quality assessment. In: Providing quality care. Ann Abor: American College of Physicians. 1989;25–69.
37. Davies BJ, Ware JE Jr. Involving consumers in quality of care assessment. Health Aff 1988;7:34–48.
38. Davis MS. Variations in patients' compliance with doctors orders, medical practice and doctor-patient interaction. Psychiatr Med 1971;2:31–54.
39. Kaplan SH. Patient reports of health status as predictors of health measures in chronic disease. J Chronic Dis 1987;40(suppl):27S–40S.
40. Vertinsky IB, Thompson WA, Uyen D. Measuring consumer desire for participation in clinical decision making. Health Serv Res 1974;9:121–134.
41. Greenfield S, Kaplan S, Ware JE Jr. Expanding patient involvement in medical care: effects on patient outcomes. Ann Intern Med 1985;102:520–528.

42. Wennberg JE, Gittelsohn A. Small area variation in healthcare delivery. Science 1973:182: 1102–1108.
43. Perrin JM, Home CJ, Berwick DM, Woolf AD, Freeman JL, Wennberg JE. Variations in rates of hospitalization of children in three urban communities. N Engl J Med 1989;320: 1183–1187.
44. Wennberg JE, Freeman JL, Culp WJ. Are hospital services rationed in New Haven or over-utilized in Boston? Lancet 1987;11:1185–1188.
45. Ellwood PM. Shattuck lecture—outcomes management, a technology of patient experience. N Engl J Med 1988;318:1549–1556.
46. Guadagnoli E, McNeil BJ. Outcomes research: hope for the future or latest rage? Inquiry 1994;31:14–34.
47. Siu AL, McGlynn EA, Morgenstern H, Brook RH. A fair approach to comparing quality of care. Health Aff 1991;10:62–75.
48. Institute of Medicine. Report of a study: a manpower policy for primary health care. Washington, DC: National Academy of Sciences, 1978.

SECTION FOUR

LEGAL IMPLICATIONS OF MANAGED CARE

CHAPTER ELEVEN

INTEGRATED PHYSICIAN ORGANIZATIONS

Alice G. Gosfield

Managed care takes multiple forms. Similarly, physician approaches to the new environment can follow a variety of models. The choice of which model makes the most sense in a given situation depends on a variety of factors ranging from the relationships among the physicians seeking to interact to the marketplace demands at a particular moment in time. Regardless of the market context in which physicians find themselves, there is no single answer regarding the right path to follow. Moreover, in the current transitional environment in which most physicians find themselves, what makes sense at one point in time may change as the market evolves or other opportunities, obstacles, or influences emerge.

This chapter addresses the range of entities into which physicians may form and the mechanisms with which physicians will typically engage along an integration continuum. The basic legal concerns associated with each are also presented. Overriding all efforts to integrate and aggregate into larger groups, however, looms the specter of antitrust law.

ANTITRUST[1]

The antitrust laws are intended to preserve free market competition in a capitalist society. Many physicians see the impact of antitrust laws, at both federal and state levels, as illogical at a minimum and certainly unfair in practice. An overview of some of the basic principles of antitrust

---

1. The author of this chapter is not an antitrust lawyer. The principles set forth here are intended to provide very basic fundamental principles and are neither comprehensive or complete. For evaluation of specific situations the advice of a health care antitrust lawyer should be obtained.

law is important to an understanding of the limits of the strategies and entities considered here.[2]

The antitrust laws protect competition, not competitors. Consequently, under the law, activities that restrict competition are seen as inimical to a free market, whereas those that increase competition are viewed favorably. Physicians often find some of the results of this approach to be counterintuitive. For example, physicians forming independent practice associations (IPAs) worry about their liability in excluding from their membership other physicians in the community. In fact, in most settings, unless an IPA has so much market share that participation is essential for a physician to practice medicine in that community, the antitrust laws view positively the creation of a competing network, which may have very exclusive or limited membership. To the antitrust regulators and enforcers, the new network contributes to competition in the marketplace.

Because of the many bases for competition in the quickly developing environment, the antitrust enforcers have announced a series of safety zones for certain behavior that they would not tend to investigate or enforce against.[3] Activities addressed include sharing information among providers regarding price and costs, aggregation of providers for the purpose of bargaining with paying entities, agreements regarding fees, sharing of information regarding price and costs from providers to payers, and joint activities among providers. It is beyond the scope of this chapter to address all of these. Physicians would be well advised to obtain legal guidance early in their strategic decision making before they undertake any joint action. It takes only two independent physicians to form a conspiracy.

Three principles should inform any joint undertaking by physicians: *(a)* never have a conversation with someone outside the bounds of your professional practice corporation or partnership that considers the subject of fees or prices, whether on a capitated (per member per month) price basis or a fee-for-service basis; *(b)* never have a conversation with someone outside the bounds of your professional practice corporation about a proposed managed care arrangement that considers whether to join or participate with a third party; and *(c)* involve an attorney who can assess the potential for antitrust risks as early as you can in your strategic considerations if you will be doing anything that involves practitioners outside your current practice arrangement.

---

2. For a lucid and straightforward presentation of antitrust principles in network formation and integration strategies written for physicians see, Ile and Lerner "Antitrust and Managed Care," *Doctors' Resource Network, American Medical Association, 1993.*
3. See "Statements of Enforcement Policy and Analytical Principles Relating to Health Care and Antitrust," U.S. Dept. of Justice and the Federal Trade Commission, Sept. 27, 1994.

ENTITIES

The entities set forth here are often identified by the acronyms associated with their names. However, the names of these organizations may change over time. For example, "group practices without walls" (GPWWs) are sometimes called "clinics without walls" (CWWs) or even "multisite group practices" (MSGPs). These are all exactly the same entities traveling under different labels. It is far more important to focus on the functions of these entities, which may, in fact, be present in a number of the structures.

Independent Practice Association (IPA)

An IPA can be the loosest form of integration among physicians. The concept is predicated upon the basic notion that the physicians involved continue to practice medicine independently in their own offices, whether they practice as solo physicians or in groups. IPAs can be single specialty (e.g., cardiology, vision care, oncology) or multispecialty (e.g., rehabilitation, primary care, or all specialties).

In terms of the form of corporate organization that can be used, these can be not-for-profit[4] (although usually not tax exempt) or profit making. They can be set up as professional corporations or as business corporations. Even in states that otherwise prohibit the corporate practice of medicine (See "Corporate Practice of Medicine," below), often, IPAs can be established as business corporations because they do not hold themselves out as practicing medicine. Rather, they just arrange for the provision of services.

If the entity is established as either a for-profit professional corporation or a business corporation, because the shareholders will hold stock in the entity, both state and federal securities laws must be considered. This can increase the expense in setting the venture in place, but it can also provide the organizers or shareholders with an opportunity to make a profit on the basis of dividends distributed to the shareholders. However, since the only revenues to an IPA come from the capitalization by the members or payment for services, frequently the generation of profits comes from dollars that would otherwise be spent on the physician members providing medical services. Where the nonprofit model is chosen, excess revenues may not be distributed to individuals, so pure profits must be used in fulfilling the purposes of the organization. The ability to get a federal tax exemption for these entities is fairly limited because they do not function for public charitable purposes, the sine qua non of federal tax exemption.

---

4. Not-for-profit means only that the profits may not be distributed in the form of dividends.

In establishing an IPA, the physicians involved have to decide not only on a governance structure, which will be expressed in the bylaws, but also on the contractual obligations of participating physicians, which are expressed in participation contracts. The participation contract serves two purposes: *(a)* it sets forth the respective obligations of the IPA and the physicians who provide services through it and *(b)* it states the basic terms upon which the IPA will enter into relationships with payers.

Typical issues to be determined in the bylaws include the size of the board and whether seats will be slotted by specialty (e.g., five primary care physicians and five specialty physicians) as well as the qualifications for membership (e.g., board certification, specific hospital staff membership, geographic location). The bylaws establish the voting rights of the physicians who are members or shareholders.

Being a member or shareholder is different from being a participating physician. Physicians can be members of an IPA network and eligible to provide services (e.g., participating physicians) without necessarily being members of the governance structure or shareholders. Shareholders need not be participating physicians, and participants need not be shareholders. These are choices groups make.

Because the participants in an IPA at any level continue to practice elsewhere, in their "outside" lives they may be offered opportunities to participate in other IPAs. One of the major decisions in the formation of an IPA is the extent of involvement in other networks the organization will permit. If the IPA determines that the physicians who are participants may not engage in managed care contracts through any mechanism other than that IPA, the IPA is considered exclusive for antitrust purposes. Under the safety zones, an exclusive IPA may not include more than 20% of the physicians of the same specialty with active staff privileges in the market area to be safe under the antitrust safe harbors.[5] In addition, although the members continue to practice independently, to avoid liability for price fixing as competitors, the regulators require that the IPA demonstrate financial risk among the participants in the form of accepting capitation payment from payers or utilizing withholds to motivate behavior. These are not the sole forms of financial risk the regulators will accept, although they are the only forms specifically identified in the safety zone statements. If an IPA is not exclusive and physicians may participate in other arrangements, then the threshold of permissible participation among like specialists rises to 30%, but the other requirements remain the same.[6]

5. See 3 at Statement 8.
6. The percentage requirements represent what is safe. If the percentages are higher, the arrangement does not necessarily violate the law, but guidance from a knowledgeable antitrust attorney should be sought.

Other issues that typically arise in the governance are what will constitute a conflict of interest or a basis for disqualification of officers or members of the board of directors. The process that will be provided to evaluate whether to terminate a member's participation is also an issue. There is real tension between the needs of the network to get rid of noncompliant physician members and the needs of the potentially excluded physician for a fair appeal. Typically, there is no legal requirement to offer a specific review process, although sometimes this matter is addressed in state law.

The major advantages of the IPA are its relative flexibility and the fact that it does not involve a total commitment from the participating physicians—they continue to practice elsewhere. Depending on the structure chosen (business corporation, professional corporation, for profit or nonprofit), they can be relatively easily formed. However, the very fact of the members' independence can be the disadvantage to these entities. Because the antitrust laws require financial integration to avoid liability among otherwise competing similar physicians, unless the organization is paid on a capitation basis or utilizes withholds, it usually can function only as a messenger of potential arrangements with payers, so each physician makes his or her own decision on whether to participate in each payer arrangement. Obviously, this is not a mechanism that can use any power of numbers to really bargain for price in the marketplace.

MSO (Medical Management/Services/Staff Organization)

An MSO can be owned entirely by physicians, solely by a hospital, by a totally separate third party, or by any combination of these. Regardless of the name, these entities perform physician office-management services. The physicians who are the customers of the MSO do not otherwise necessarily relate to each other. They are in independent practice but managed, often by common principles established through contracts. Frequently the MSO provides basic office-management services including secretarial and reception services, billing and collection, group purchasing, and computer services. The relationship is established on the basis of a contract between the physician (or physician group) and the MSO.

MSOs sometimes offer a menu of services to physicians and physician groups. Sometimes they actually purchase the assets of physician practices and then manage them. When this approach is taken, all of the basic legal aspects of the commercial transaction of the purchase must be addressed. For example, if real estate is part of the assets, for the physicians to continue to practice at their original location there will have to be a lease between the MSO and the physician practice. Often these transactions entail very long-term management contracts. When outside entrepreneurial entities form the MSO, these organizations bring to bear for the physician practice increased capital and, presumably, management expertise.

Some of these organizations also incorporate some IPA functions, performing as negotiators of managed care contracts for their physician customers, usually on a messenger model. In some models, though, the various physician customer entities are combined into a loosely amalgamated network to negotiate contracts for their members.

When these organizations are owned by physicians, there are antitrust concerns involving the potential for otherwise competing physicians to fix prices, engage in group boycotts of managed care entities, or allocate markets. Consequently, whether owned solely by physicians or by physicians in combination with others, antitrust may be an issue along with certain Medicare fraud and abuse problems (see "Fraud and Abuse," below).

The major virtue of the MSO is that it removes from the physicians responsibility for those aspects of practice with which the physicians are least comfortable. In many deals, this value is joined with offering the physician customers access to capital. The disadvantages are that once the physician's assets are owned by someone else, the basic inputs into his or her ability to provide clinical services is in play. If the MSO and the physician disagree about what is necessary or appropriate, it can directly influence clinical care.

Access to capital has been widely trumpeted as necessary for physician strategic success. This may be true for large group practices that are themselves seeking to integrate or acquire a large number of other groups or for entities that are seeking to control global capitation for a large number of lives. Smaller physician practices do not necessarily need real capital and may be able to contract from others for what they need in terms of computer services and systems that facilitate managing the practice.

Multisite Group Practice (MSGP)

MSGPs have been marketed to physicians as integration with autonomy. They are often created under the jurisdiction of new state laws permitting limited-liability corporations or partnerships. The concept of the group practice without walls is that previously independent physicians join together into one economic unit without leaving their previous practice locations, while maintaining a certain degree of economic independence.

The limited-liability corporations permit to corporations the same tax advantages enjoyed by partnerships. In addition, unlike subchapter S corporations under federal tax laws, these laws do not limit the permissible number of shareholders. In many states, they allow corporations themselves to be shareholders (although in some states only licensed physicians may be shareholders for professional practice even in these new corporations). However, not all MSGPs are limited-liability corporations.

Whatever legal structure is selected, these entities require all the same mechanisms and conceptual underpinnings as a fully integrated group practice merger, such as shareholder or partnership agreements, employment agreements, buy-sell agreements, bylaws, and restrictive covenants. How to value capitalization and bring it into the new entity is always an issue. In addition, because of the Medicare statutes, these entities must demonstrate sufficient integration to meet a number of reimbursement and fraud-and-abuse tests (see "Medicare Reimbursement Issues" and "Fraud and Abuse," below). Further, without sufficient financial integration, these organizations do not protect the participating physicians from the antitrust laws. In this author's opinion, when the emphasis is on maintaining autonomy, this type of entity works in very few situations and is more illusory than real as an option.

Full Integration

Full physician integration entails the creation of a unitary physician practice entity, usually in the form of a professional corporation or partnership that is the sole mechanism through which the involved physicians provide professional services. The physicians themselves are usually employees of the entity, and some or all are also shareholders or partners.

These practice entities are usually created through merger or acquisition. The only difference between this approach and the MSGP is the extent of economic and operational autonomy at disparate practice locations. Common issues to be addressed include valuation of the assets brought to the table by the prospective partners and all of the traditional issues associated with forming a group, such as percentage of ownership and the basis for its determination, restrictive covenants, and buy-sell and shareholders agreements. In addition, since hard assets are at issue, including practice locations, real estate concerns are often on the table, too.

The primary virtue in full physician practice integration is that if structured appropriately, it eliminates the antitrust and fraud-and-abuse problems typically encountered in the other mechanisms. The disadvantage is that it is like a marriage. Once you enter into such an arrangement, you have made a very major commitment from which it is very difficult to extricate yourself legally and practically.

Physician-Hospital Organizations (PHOs)

PHOs combine a hospital (or several hospitals in some models) with a selected group of physicians—usually from the hospital medical staff—into a new entity that offers the services of both in a one-stop-shopping approach. Although many PHOs hope to get bundled or capitated payments from payers, most start off with separate hospital-physician payments. The structuring is similar to that of an IPA, with bylaws for the PHO and provider-participation agreements for both the hospital as a provider and the physicians.

There are two essential models: *(a)* individual physicians become members of the PHO directly through participation agreements, and some are selected to participate in the organization's governance; or *(b)* the physicians form an IPA that contracts with its members, and the IPA contracts with the PHO to, in effect, deliver a network of practitioners unto the PHO. The IPA model is somewhat more expensive because it entails yet another corporation with all the expenses of administration, taxes, and management associated with any IPA (although often in a limited way); but it sometimes has the option of contracting outside the PHO context as well. The IPA model gives the physicians a mechanism through which they can consider PHO-related issues apart from the hospital personnel who sit on the PHO board. In the non-IPA model, the physicians have no place to obtain separate legal advice regarding the activities of the organization, and there is no structure other than the bylaws of the PHO that determines how the physicians interrelate.

Whichever model is selected, the primary mechanism of governance is to give the participants (physicians and hospital) a fully equal say in the structure of the entity. However, if the organization is established as a tax-exempt entity, the IRS regulators have taken the position that no more than 20% of the board of director positions may be held by physicians, because of rules against private inurement. For physicians, this seriously undermines the appeal of a tax-exempt PHO. Still, there will be circumstances in some communities where physicians will want to proceed, nonetheless.

Regardless of the model, the primary reason to form a PHO is in the belief that a new organization will change the way both the hospital and the physicians do business and make each more attractive than either would be alone. For the physicians, some of the virtues include the energy, capital and expertise the hospital can bring to bear. By the same token, however, when the physicians defer to the hospital or fail to stay as active as they initially intended, the hospital position on various issues may become dominant.

The reason for a physician to join a PHO is to gain access to the business the PHO will have. The volume of business any physician will obtain depends on his/her type of practice and the success of the PHO. For physicians who are afraid to enter into the managed care fray with both feet, the PHO provides a very limited way to begin to learn about managed care. For the members of the medical staff in general, the PHO structure also changes fundamentally the power relationship between the hospital and the medical staff: In the traditional medical staff structure, the physicians are underpaid, highly trained, technical advisors on issues of quality and credentialing to the board of directors, which retains all of the legal authority for the decisions on which the physicians provide input. In the PHO, the hospital and physicians directly share the governance of the organization. The physicians have just as much right to inquire about the bona fides of the hospital in seeking to meet the needs of the new organization as the hospital representatives do to inquire about the physicians' activities. The physician board members, like the hospital representatives, are fiduciaries to the PHO and must navigate the tension between their responsibility to the PHO and their individual interests. The physicians who join a PHO remain independent in the rest of their practices. This is the polar opposite of the next model.

Hospital Employment

It is increasingly common for hospitals or their affiliated practice organizations to employ previously independent physicians directly. These employment relationships are exactly that; they entail all the traditional indicia of employment: the employer tells the employee how, when, where, and at what charge to provide services. In some states, because of the corporate practice of medicine doctrine (see "Corporate Practice of Medicine," below), the employment mechanism is through an affiliated physician-practice corporation that is controlled by a physician employee of the hospital.

The primary value in the employment model is the virtual removal of the physician from any management aspects of the practice. He or she functions at the direction and instruction of the employer. When the employer is also buying the assets of the physician's prior practice, all of the problems associated with MSO asset purchases arise as well. These include valuation, employment of ancillary clinical personnel, control over management of the practice location, and pay-out terms. Fraud-and-abuse issues also arise in these transactions because whichever entity actually purchases the assets and whichever actually employs the physician, the hospital ultimately benefits in some way (see "Fraud and Abuse," below). In academic medical centers, these issues are somewhat less troublesome, since the teaching mission is a predominant concern. When the physician joins a faculty practice plan or its equivalent, the benefit to the hospital of referrals is often a secondary issue. Still, these matters are relatively unresolved under the fraud-and-abuse laws and bear consideration by a knowledgeable health lawyer in every transaction because the current fraud-and-abuse environment is so dynamic and volatile.

Other

In some constructs, an academic medical center or a large tertiary care institution decides to form an integrated delivery system. This mechanism incorporates a number of the features discussed. The basic idea is to create a "seamless web" of care delivery through a broad continuum of services, bringing the physicians intimately into the structure. Mature versions of such organizations do exist. For example, Intermountain Health in Salt Lake City and the Henry Ford Health System in Detroit are long-standing integrated systems that even include their own managed care entities in addition to physician and ancillary service integration.

Most of the systems that are developing today, however, are far from seamless and quite evolutionary. Within many of these aggregations one can find employment relationships, MSOs, PHOs, MSGPs, IPAs, and independent integrated physician groups all relating in various degrees of affinity. Often, within the nonprofit setting, a tax-exempt organization in support of the integrating entity will be formed in a foundation model of group practice. For the physicians, the tax-exempt nature of these entities can limit compensation, undermine certain retirement benefits, and truncate governance opportunities. For most of the markets around the country, it will be many years before the true value and success of these IDS structures will be susceptible to evaluation.

Finally, another acronym that is frequently discussed among physicians is the PO, or physician organization. The term is vague, with no defined parameters. Generally speaking, this term is used to describe a physician-controlled entity that may employ some physicians, contract with others, offer MSO services to some or all, and take capitation dollars from payers for whom they manage virtually all the care. In some settings in the most evolved managed care markets, this entails "global capitation" in which the physicians get 85% of the premium dollar collected by the HMO (for example) and are then responsible for contracting for and arranging for all of the care for the populations for which the plan contracts with the PO. The structure of these entities is fluid, and whatever the group selects or whatever evolves over time can be accommodated within the rubric. Generally speaking, the term is used to describe a physician-controlled entity that is fairly high up on the food chain of integration and, in the most successful models, can ultimately evolve into its own HMO or licensed managed care entity.

LEGAL ISSUES

The creation of any of the integrated structures will require legal documents; the operation of any will also create ongoing legal concerns. One of the first issues for physicians forming or participating in the governance of any of these entities is liability insurance for both the directors and the entity itself. Unless the integrating entity will practice as a professional provider, in most instances this is not malpractice insurance but coverage for general liability and for the special activities that are essential to one of the integrating structures.

In addition, board members will want to be sure the bylaws establish that the organization will indemnify them for any liabilities they may incur as a result of their duly authorized activities on behalf of the entity for which they have undertaken fiduciary responsibility by participating on the board. Sometimes, particularly in less integrated modes such as IPAs and MSGPs (depending on whether they are established as professional corporations that hold themselves out as actually providing care), they may need regular malpractice insurance too, to protect against liability for bad outcomes in the actual delivery of care.

Corporate Practice of Medicine

In many states,[7] long-standing legal doctrines establish that physicians may not be employed by anyone other than a professional of similar licensure. This principle is based on the public policy that the essence of a professional is to exercise independent judgment in the practice of the profession. To be employed by a business corporation would put the professional under the direction of an unlicensed individual who is in a master-servant relationship (in legal terms) with the professional. In those states that prohibit the corporate practice of medicine, physicians may only be employed by a professional corporation, partnership, or another professional.[8] Professional corporations, which provide the limited liability of the business corporate structure for commercial aspects of their business, do not shield the participants from malpractice liability for their professional judgments.

In some integration models, then, nonprofessionals, including hospital administrators, insurance companies, and others, must establish affiliated professional corporations that are captives of their activities by virtue of having the shares of the professional corporation held by an employee of the corporation (e.g., medical director) who does not necessarily practice medicine through the primary business structure. Another approach is to put nonphysician affiliates of the integrating entity onto the board of the

---

7. See, Jacobson "Prohibition Against Corporate Practice of Medicine: Dinosaur or Dynamic Doctrine," *1993 Health Law Handbook*, Clark Boardman Callaghan, New York, ppP 67–98.
8. In some states, there is an exception for employment by hospitals or by nonprofit entities.

captive professional entity. Depending on the degree of control sought by the integrating entity (including MSOs and hospitals), the professional corporation may function as one in name only, although the law will require that the board may be ousted by the shareholders. If none of the employed physicians is a shareholder, however, the result is the same as if the physicians were employed by the business entity.

Medicare Reimbursement Issues

In many markets where integration is at the forefront of physician strategic thinking in the face of burgeoning managed care programs, the Medicare fee-for-service segment of the market remains strong.[9] Many of the motivations and purposes of integration run at cross-purposes with the major concerns of both the Medicare reimbursement rules as well as Medicare fraud-and-abuse laws. Although integration is based on one-stop shopping that layers providers and practitioners, Medicare seeks direct relationships with its providers. Medicare does not recognize IPAs as entities eligible for Medicare payment. Multisite group practices are recognized only if they are sufficiently integrated to have the ancillary clinical personnel employed by the same entity as the physician who would submit claims incorporating their services.

Two basic Medicare principles get in the way of the new operations:

1. Medicare will pay for those services that are performed personally by a physician or that are an integral, although incidental, part of the physician's personal professional service to a patient. This standard has three components, which are set forth in the Carrier's Manual (the book that tells the Medicare Part B carrier how to administer the program): (*a*) the ancillary clinical personnel must be the W-2 employee of the claiming physician practice; (*b*) a physician member of the group must be on the premises and immediately available to assist ancillary personnel during all times that they are performing services included in the physician's charge; and (*c*) there must be a physician service to which the ancillary services are incidental.[10] Based on these rules, the use of midlevel practitioners (e.g., nurse practitioners, physicians assistants, CRNAs) is seriously undermined in the Medicare program, and the organizational interrelationships that make these individuals available are limited.

9. For more information about Medicare reimbursement for physicians generally see Gosfield, "Unintentional Part B False Claims Pitfalls for the Unwary," *1993 Health Law Handbook*, Clark Boardman Callaghan, pp 205–230.
10. Carrier's Manual §2050.

2. The right to receive Medicare payment belongs to the beneficiary, who may then assign that right to a physician. The physician may choose to accept assignment. Physicians who agree to accept assignment 100% of the time are "participating physicians." The physician who accepts assignment may only "reassign" his or her right to payment in limited circumstances adopted as part of the Medicare Anti-Fraud and Abuse Amendments of 1977. These rules have recently been further limited, which creates additional problems.

Payment may be made to the physician's direct employer, to an inpatient facility, or to a free-standing outpatient clinic for services provided there.[11] Consequently, independent contractor arrangements are limited, and payment to MSOs or IPAs are not recognized at all. Under a Medicare risk contract with an HMO, some of these problems go away, but they are real obstacles to integration in mixed arrangements, which most physicians must address to avoid problems.

Fraud and Abuse

In addition to reimbursement requirements, Medicare and Medicaid prohibitions against kickbacks and certain designated referrals seriously impede a number of integration strategies. The two fundamental federal laws at issue are the antikickback prohibitions, which pertain to all Medicare and Medicaid transactions and all participants in them, and the Stark II amendment, which pertains only to physician referrals and then only for a specified list of "designated health services."

Under the so-called Stark II law,[12] a physician may not refer a Medicare or (Medicaid) patient to an entity with which he or she has a financial interest when the referral is for certain designated health services,[13] unless the referral meets one of some approximately 17 statutory exceptions. The statute is subject to regulatory interpretation. Partial, initial regulations were published 14 August 1995. Because they are incomplete they make compliance difficult at best.

The law is so broadly drafted that referrals include intragroup referrals. There are a number of exceptions that take into account certain physician group-practice arrangements, but these are available only if the "group"

---

11. Carrier's Manual §3060.
12. 42 USC §1395nn et seq.
13. The designated services are clinical laboratory services, physical therapy services, occupational therapy services, radiology including MRI, CT, and ultrasound, radiation therapy services and supplies, durable medical equipment and supplies, parenteral and enteral nutrients, equipment and supplies, prosthetics, orthotics and prosthetic devices and supplies, home health services, outpatient prescription drugs and inpatient and outpatient hospital services. (42 USC §1395nn(h)(6))

meets the statutory definition of one, which is quite narrow and very much limits autonomy within groups. For example, among the eight requirements for qualifying as a group, substantially all of the services of members of the group must be provided through the group and each member of the group must provide through the group substantially the full range of services he or she provides. In addition, the services must be claimed under a single group-provider number.

The law specifically addresses compensation formulas, both within groups and as part of employment relationships. In neither setting may the physician be rewarded for his or her volume of referrals (defined as any request for a service, item, or good payable under Part B). The law does say the physician may be paid under the employment exception directly for his or her own productivity and under the group practice definition on a productivity bonus that may include profit sharing or services provided "incident to" his or her own services.

Because Stark II financial relationships include compensation as well as ownership and because designated services include inpatient and outpatient hospital services, transactions that entail hospital-affiliated integration must be carefully evaluated. At a minimum, financing of a new entity such as a PHO, MSO, or IPA by the hospital with disproportionate return to the integrated physicians would raise issues under both Stark II and the antikickback statute.

The Stark II law establishes a direct prohibition. Both the prohibited referral and the submission of a claim by the referred-to entity are punishable by a $15,000 civil money penalty and even by a $100,000 penalty for a scheme to circumvent the statute. If the arrangement cannot meet the Stark II exceptions, there is no point in proceeding. Even if the arrangement can qualify, a separate provision in law must still be taken into account.

The antikickback law[14] is a broader statute, but it has been interpreted in safe harbor regulations that address those transactions that may tend to induce referrals but do not violate the law.[15]

Practice purchases, whether by physicians or others, present their own set of issues, since they are addressed in Stark II and the safe harbors. The safe harbor regulations have specifically raised the legitimacy of hospitals buying physician practices outright. The only explicitly safe purchase is that by one physician of a retiring physician's practice, and the deal must be concluded no later than 1 year from the date of the agreement of sale. Therefore, many deals are structured as asset purchases on the theory that

---

14. 42 USC §1320a-7(b)
15. 42 CFR §1001.952 et seq.

the integration regulators never defined a "practice." Even so, points of vulnerability include valuation of the practice, payment over time, and payment for goodwill. Each of these should be carefully reviewed by knowledgeable health care counsel. The Stark II provision that pertains is one for a one-time "isolated transaction." Regualtions under Stark do not allow payments over any time period.

Special State Laws

Besides these federal laws, increasingly, states are adopting their own antireferral legislation as well as "anti–managed care" legislation. A good number of states also have state antitrust laws. Each must be considered in the context of each transaction, as well. "Any willing provider" legislation may undermine the ability of a network to exclude undesirable physicians. Regulation of utilization-review entities may require review and approval by a state agency prior to beginning to make utilization management decisions. Offering discounted rates to groups such as purchasers who are not themselves directly regulated as HMOs or insurance companies can require qualification as a PPO under state law. Many states are now also considering regulating PHOs, because the advent of global capitation strategies raises issues about the financial viability of the entities taking financial risk, since defined populations must get their care from those entities. If these organizations fail, large numbers of patients may lose their access to health care services. State health reform initiatives generate additional legal issues.

Operational Issues

The purpose of most integration strategies is to demonstrate to purchasers the value the integrated entity will bring to those who would seek to do business with them. The essence of value is controlled costs, using high-quality processes, and producing good outcomes for patients, as demonstrated in data.[16] A variety of activities essential to integration success raise other legal issues.

CREDENTIALING

The first step to producing value is selecting a group of coproviders who can adhere to the demands of the integrated structure. Besides the an-

---

16. For a discussion of data issues and other measures of value, see Gosfield, "Measuring Performance and Quality: The State of the Art and Legal Concerns," *1995 Health Law Handbook*, Clark Boardman Callaghan, pp 31–68.

titrust issues already considered, there is additional legal liability in the physician selection and retention decisions of integrated organizations. Increasingly, the case law is holding managed care organizations liable for the bad outcomes that result to their patients from some of their decisions. Based on notions of ostensible agency ("you held this person out to the public as your representative") and negligent credentialing ("the patient would not have been harmed but for your selecting this provider and limiting patient choice to those you selected"), the process by which physicians are chosen and retained within groups and networks raises its own concerns.

The national practitioner data bank is one source of information about potential participants in any venture. Its resources are available to anyone who both provides care and has an organized peer review mechanism. Even if a group chooses not to access the data bank directly, it is wise to get physicians to provide copies of their data bank profiles for evaluation prior to affiliation with them.

Profiling physicians within integrated structures to identify both good performers from whom to learn as well as those who need additional attention or separation from the group is an essential feature of a credentialing policy.[17] Procedures for review and mechanisms of rereview should be reduced to writing and followed. The worst liability comes when an organization claims to offer these types of safeguards and then either does not provide them or does not adhere to established procedures.

Utilization Management Liability

The second special form of liability that may fall on integrated structures is that which arises from managing utilization. Again, case law on this issue is scarce, but we are beginning to see an allocation of liability among the attending physician and the managed care organization and its components (e.g., utilization review contractor) for utilization management judgments. Use of clinical practice guidelines and prior authorization for certain services are common techniques of management.[18]

Selection of standards, procedures for making decisions, and mechanisms of appeal are also essential aspects of a utilization management policy for an integrating entity. For the physician who is participating in these

---

17. For a discussion of issues in developing a credentialing policy see, Gosfield, "PPO Credentialing Policies: Legal Concerns and Practical Guidelines," *AAPPO Journal*, Vol. 3, No 5, (Oct 1993), pp 19–26.

18. For more information on guidelines, their uses and applications see, Gosfield, "Clinical Practice Guidelines and the Law: Applications and Implications," *1994 Health Law Handbook*, Clark Boardman Callaghan, pp 65–99.

organizations, appeal of decisions with which he or she disagrees is important. By the same token, knowledge of and documentation of deviation from the established standards are legal concerns too.

Incentive Structures

To motivate the production of value on behalf of the organization, physician financial incentives are frequently used. In their most basic forms, under fee-for-service, productivity bonuses have been used to reward physicians who work harder. In a managed care setting, the incentives are reversed. Under a capitation system, providing fewer services is the financial goal. While it is not the purpose of this chapter to consider incentive payment techniques, it is important to note that incentive structures do have legal implications.

Under federal law, programs that motivate physicians to provide less service must conform with Medicare mandates that prohibit underutilization and premature discharge. In addition, depending on where the incentive lies, under some state regulatory schemes acceptance of risk that creates incentives requires additional agency scrutiny and requirements to comply with state statutes. Finally, the interrelationship between the managed care goals and the Medicare system must be carefully evaluated in structuring transactions. Often, physicians will assume that if they do not include Medicare patients in their incentive payment formulas, the law cannot reach their transaction. This is inaccurate. The relevant relationships must be reviewed in their totality.

CONCLUSION

Physician integration models are burgeoning, and hybrids are emerging as the marketplace changes. Although this chapter has focused primarily on structuring and its legal issues, the success of any physician integration activity will depend not on the boxes and arrows through which it functions, but in the operational reality of its performance and the extent to which it can produce the value purchasers seek. Although legal issues are important, they should inform the choice of structure but not dominate the approach. The real challenge for physicians will not be structure but clinical results and outcomes measured against the new marketplace demands.

By the same token, however, in obtaining legal advice, it is critical to turn to lawyers with a track record on these issues. Although it will be difficult for a lawyer to point to significant longitudinal success with any of the new entities, at a minimum the physicians' representative should be both fully conversant with the range of issues that will arise and willing to get specialty help (e.g., antitrust, tax, or ERISA counselors, as necessary). Many physician organizations (e.g., the American Medical Association, American Academy of Family Physicians, American College of Physicians, state medical societies, and specialty organizations) have begun to develop networks of consultants and lawyers who have been evaluated with regard to their asserted bona fides regarding these types of representations. Physicians should be careful and aggressive in selecting their advisers, regardless of the strategy they select.

CHAPTER TWELVE

MANAGED CARE: THE LEGAL IMPLICATIONS

Christopher E. Nolin and Christopher G. Lang

Managed care has resulted in a profusion of new business forms, new legal disputes, and new legal theories, each having ramifications throughout the health care world and raising a host of legal issues. Legal commentary in this area is accumulating at astounding speed, and the lists of legal implications continue to multiply and change, even as managed care itself expands and develops.

As a result, a full catalog of managed care legal issues is beyond the scope of any single chapter. Nevertheless, from the individual physician's perspective, there are several defined areas of legal conflict that are of primary importance. These include malpractice implications, major issues raised by managed care contracts, and government regulation in the areas of antifraud and antitrust law. This chapter discusses each of these topics separately, although the overlap between them is extensive.

MALPRACTICE IN THE ERA OF MANAGED CARE

Over the past hundred years, the American health care system has undergone many significant changes,[1] moving from a home-based system to a hospital-based system, from a focus on nursing care to one on high technology, and from a system that was patient-driven to one that was physician-driven and in turn to one that is increasingly payor-driven.[2] Operat-

---

1. *See* P. Torrens, Historical Evolution and Overview of Health Services in the United States, in Introduction to Health Services 3 (Stephen J. Williams & Paul R. Torrens, eds. 1980).
2. *See* V. Randall, Managed Care, Utilization Review, and Financial Risk Shifting: Compensating Patients for Health Care Cost Containment Injuries, 17 Puget Sound L. Rev. 1, 9 (1993). As used in this chapter, the term "payor" includes any third-party paying entity including insurance companies and managed care organizations.

ing within this new system can be difficult for physicians who long have been the sole medical advisers to their patients regarding medical care. Now, case managers who are not the patients' physicians are making financial and medical decisions that can contradict and even override the physicians' advice. Physicians must become fluent in this new system and learn how to practice medicine effectively within it.

Notwithstanding the managed care health systems in place today, a physician's duty to his or her patient remains paramount. As has been true for centuries, physicians above all else must care for their patients, acting as their fiduciary and standing up for them against all others to ensure that they receive appropriate medical care.

Under past fee-for-service reimbursement arrangements, it was relatively simple for a physician to treat patients based solely on the medical effectiveness of the treatments, with little regard for cost. Those days, however, are fast drawing to a close. Under many current reimbursement plans, most notably those involving managed care organizations (MCOs), a physician is constantly forced to consider (either consciously or unconsciously) the costs of care in making treatment decisions. The consequences of incurring "excess" costs may be catastrophic. If the physician is capitated, overspending may be financially ruinous. If an MCO is footing the bill, the physician may be fired, "deselected," or "decredentialed." Because access to patients and facilities may depend on MCO affiliations, exclusion from the MCO could end a physician's career. Operating within the restrictive MCO environment, therefore, can be very difficult for physicians, whose duty to their patients remains unchanged.

At the same time, in malpractice cases, physicians are regularly excoriated for failing to do "everything reasonably possible" to obtain a good result. Although this is not the legal standard of care, a jury faced with a severely injured person is unlikely to respond well to the argument that treatment was not "cost effective." The physician who pays too much attention to the economics of practice may find out too late that there must be good medical, not economic, reasons to justify a course of action.

Thus, it is important for physicians to be aware of their state's malpractice legal standards and to understand how operating within the MCO environment will require extra caution by a physician so as to avoid increased malpractice liability exposure.

A Physician's Legal Duty to Patients

Ethical guidelines promulgated by medical associations,[3] internal moral value systems, and the law all affect how physicians views their duty to

---

3. *See, e.g.,* American Medical Association's Code of Ethics.

their patients. While ethics and morals are vital to a physician's practice and sense of purpose, it is the legal definition of duty that forms the basis of malpractice actions.[4]

Under current legal principles, a physician's duty to his or her patient is established in accordance with the appropriate legal "standard of care."[5] A physician who can convince a jury that a patient has been treated within this standard of care should not be liable for malpractice, regardless of the outcome of the physician's care.[6] The basic working definition is the degree of skill and care that a reasonably competent physician would apply in similar circumstances.[7] Unfortunately, applying this standard of care is more difficult than it appears, both for physicians and for the courts.

To define this standard of care at trial, both sides typically offer expert testimony from physicians about what the general practice is with respect to the care at issue. After both sides have argued their cases, the trier of fact, usually a jury, weighs the available testimony and determines (a) what it believes is the appropriate standard and (b) whether the defendant physician followed this standard. In most states, as long as the trier of fact determines that the physician followed what a respectable minority of competent physicians would have done under the circumstances, then the physician has not breached the duty of care to the patient.[8]

Under this system, with every malpractice action, the trier of fact redefines the standard of care. No set of specific medical procedures always falls within it, and therefore it becomes difficult for physicians to know prospectively whether their practices conform to the standard of care. Furthermore, the definition of standard of care is fluid, not only changing over time, but also narrowing and widening over the course of treating a patient.

The standard of care can be analogized to a river,[9] and this helps to clarify exactly what the concept entails. In caring for a patient, a physician moves down the river. As the physician rows downstream, each stroke

---

4. This is not meant to understate the importance of ethical guidelines or internal values, either as they affect the practice of medicine of their impact on juries in malpractice cases.
5. *See Hall v. Hilbun*, 466 So. 2d 856 (Miss. 1985).
6. In order to establish a prima facie case of medical malpractice, a plaintiff needs to show that (1) the physician owed the patient a duty of due care, (2) the physician breached that duty to the patient, (3) the patient suffered an injury which was proximately caused by the breach, and (4) injury is one for which the patient can be compensated. *See* W. Page Keeton et al., *Prosser and Keeton on the Law of Torts*, (5th ed. 1984) (hereinafter Prosser on Torts), Section 30.
7. *See* Prosser on Torts, supra note 6, Section 32.
8. *See*, e.g., *Chumbler v. McClure*, 505 F.2d 489, 492 (6th Cir. 1974) ("Where two or more schools of thought exist . . . each of which is supported by responsible medical authority, it is not malpractice to be among the minority in a given city who follow one of the accepted schools").
9. Credit for the river analogy goes to Professor Francis Miller of the Boston University School of Law who uses it effectively in her health law lectures.

taken (e.g., each diagnosis and treatment decision) must fall within the banks of the river. As the river widens in certain areas, the physician is given latitude in choosing what approach to take (there may be several different tests or procedures available, any one of which is acceptable). In other instances, there are only one or two narrow options available if the physician is to stay within the standard of care. Finally, as rivers change their course over the years, so too the standard of care constantly shifts. As medical knowledge and technology develop, the standard of care gradually incorporates what is discovered, and physicians are held to the newer standard. What was considered appropriate one year, may become outdated only a few months later.[10] Physicians, therefore, are required to remain well-informed about the latest advances in their field, so that when appropriate, they can be incorporated in the physicians' normal treatment regimens.[11]

With each jury in each case having to redefine this fluid standard, juries over a series of cases express considerable variation in their definitions. Since the individual physician cannot know this definition with precision beforehand, the overall incentive for the physician is to render the most thorough care possible, to avoid the possibility of liability.

The traditional fee-for-service arrangement did not counterbalance this incentive. It was, in large part, a two-person relationship (physician and patient). When an MCO is involved, a new triangle of relationships is formed. First, the MCO and the patient enter into a contractual relationship wherein limited services and procedures are offered to the patient in exchange for a certain dollar amount. Second, the MCO and the physician enter into a contractual relationship that carries with it its own set of risks and benefits for the physician.[12] Third, the patient chooses a physician under the MCO plan, and they enter into a contractual relationship, with the physician agreeing to treat the patient in accordance with his or her legal duty as a physician. This new dynamic can create conflicts of loyalty for the physician working within the MCO framework.

Cost-cutting Techniques of MCOs

Since MCOs are designed to reduce health care costs, their existence is inexorably tied to their success in limiting the amount of medical services provided to members. To accomplish this goal, MCOs employ a number

10. *See* E. B. Hirshfeld, Should Ethical and Legal Standards For Physicians Be Changed To Accommodate New Models For Rationing Health Care, 140 U. Penn. L. Rev. 1809 (1992).
11. *See* R. N. Pearson, The Role of Custom in Medical Malpractice Cases, 51 Ind. L. J. 528, 538–557 (1976).
12. *See* discussion on physician contracting with MCOs, this chapter.

of cost-cutting techniques.[13] Two commonly employed cost-cutting strategies are utilization review and financial risk shifting, both of which can affect a physician's legal duty to his or her patients.

Utilization review (UR) consists of determining, either retrospectively, prospectively, or concurrently, if certain medical services are appropriate, often defined as "medically necessary."[14] If the service requested is not considered medically necessary, then the MCO will not pay for it.[15] UR can be conducted by MCOs directly, by MCO physicians, or by independent agencies hired by the MCO. In any case, the UR reviewer usually examines the patient's records and compares the requested services with statistical norms developed from large sample surveys in determining if the service is medically necessary. Physicians and caregivers who also act as UR reviewers for their own or each other's patients have little incentive to reduce health care costs. Therefore, MCOs frequently relegate UR to non-care-giving personnel or to outside agencies. By having MCO administrative personnel or a hired organization conduct the UR, however, the function of cutting costs is displaced from the actual care of the patient. Thus, there is an increased likelihood that necessary and appropriate services might be inadvertently denied.[16] As discussed below, physicians must be careful of the effect that UR has on their medical decision making, to ensure that loyalty to the patient is maintained.

The second cost-cutting mechanism common to MCOs is financial risk shifting. Under this concept, MCOs attempt to affect physician behavior by shifting the financial loss of certain decision making from the MCO to the physician. There are a number of ways to accomplish this, all of which are based on some form of bonus or punishment scheme for the physician.[17] Among the most frequently used forms of financial risk shifting are capitation structures (set payment per enrollee), withholding (retaining a percentage of payment to reward or punish use trends at year-end), per

13. In addition, MCOs, viewing their members as a single collective entity, structure programs around what is best for the group as a whole. MCOs spend significant health care dollars in preventive medicine and wellness programs, attempting to improve the overall health of their members while reducing the number of patients requiring more expensive acute care procedures.
14. For a detailed discussion of utilization review techniques, *see* U.S. Gen. Accounting Office, Pub. No. HRD-93–22FS, Utilization Review: Information on External Review Organizations, at 8–9 (1992).
15. Under retrospective UR review, the determination regarding payment is made after the procedure/test has been performed. Therefore, if payment is denied, either the patient must pay for the services out of pocket or the doctor must absorb the cost. In a prospective or concurrent UR system, reimbursement decisions are made before the medical service is provided. The patient is then presented with the choice of going ahead with the procedure, knowing it is not covered by the MCO, or opting for a different course of treatment which would be reimbursed. *See* R. A. Hinden, and A. L. Elden, Liability Issues for Managed Care Entities, 14 Seton Hall Legis. J. 1 (1990).
16. *See* L. L. Kloss, Quality Review and Utilization Management, in The New Healthcare Market 680, 684 (Peter Boland ed., 1988).
17. *See* A. L. Hillman, Financial Incentives for Physicians in HMOs: Is There a Conflict of Interest?, 317 N. Engl. J. Med. 1743 (1987).

diem payments (flat fee per day per patient), and physician profit sharing.[18]

Regardless of the specific financial-risk-shifting program used, subject physicians are faced with a strong financial incentive to reduce the overall amount of medical services provided to their patients.[19] As with UR programs, the key issue for a physician working under a risk-shifting program is how to keep the level of medical care low enough to be profitable and yet high enough for the patient to receive appropriate care.

Physician Malpractice Risks in the MCO Environment

The overarching goal of all managed care systems is to provide quality health care to all members while simultaneously controlling costs. To accomplish this, MCOs operate under the belief that providing a given level of service for every patient requires that certain limitations on the extent of covered services be incorporated into medical decision making. At times, this control over physician practice comes into conflict with traditional notions of medical care, as well as with the physician's own medical opinions. It is in these areas of turbulence—where a physician and an MCO are in disagreement—that the physician runs the greater risk of assuming additional malpractice liabilities.

A physician's undivided loyalty to a patient is recognized as the cornerstone of American health care. Without confidence in this loyalty, patients would be hesitant about going to their physicians and openly discussing their medical concerns.[20] Moreover, many Americans believe that equal access to health care is a fundamental right.[21] With these concepts in mind, it is not surprising that some commentators have suggested that MCOs are violating the ethical underpinnings of American health care by enticing physicians to alter their medical practices in response to cost-cutting techniques.[22] The strength of the public's belief in access and its scorn for limitations on care forced by economics in individual cases is exemplified in the notorious case of *Fox v. Health Net of California*.[23] In that case, the plaintiff had advanced breast cancer and was identified by specialist physicians as a

---

18. *See* Randall, supra note 2, at 31 and sources cited.
19. This is in direct contrast to the traditional fee-for-service arrangements in which physicians have a financial incentive to overutilize services.
20. A. M. Capron, Containing Health Care Costs: Ethical and Legal Implications of Changes in the Methods of Paying Physicians, 36 Case W. Res. L. Rev. 708 (1986).
21. *See* K. R. Wing, The Right to Health Care, 2 Annals Health L. 161 (1993).
22. *See* Randall, supra note 2, at 37; J. J. Frankel, Medical Malpractice Law and Health Care Cost Containment: Lessons for Reformers from the Clash of Cultures, 103 Yale L.J. 1297 (1994).
23. The description of the *Fox* case is borrowed from G. T. Schwartz, National Health Care Reform or Trial: A National Health Care Program: What its Effect Would be on American Tort Law and Malpractice Law, 79 Cornell L. Rev. 1339, 1371 (1994) and sources cited.

candidate for a bone marrow transplant. From the HMO's point of view, the procedure would have been very expensive, and its efficacy for breast cancer patients was unproven. When her HMO refused to preapprove the procedure, she was eventually able to raise funds elsewhere. She died less than a year after the transplant, but before her death she filed suit against the HMO. The jury awarded her $12 million in compensatory damages and $77 million in punitive damages.[24] Among other things, the plaintiff's attorney suggested that the medical director who made the decision might have anticipated a bonus based upon his control of costs for the plaintiff's group. Although the case was not aimed at a treating physician, it graphically illustrates the violent reaction juries can have to "economic" arguments.

While there is no escaping the conflict between cutting costs and providing adequate patient care, *Fox* stands out not only because of the size of the verdict but also because relatively few cases have been reported in which this conflict is discussed. Physicians are left with little guidance as they determine how to ensure adequate care while operating within an MCO environment.

The seminal case discussing MCO cost cutting and malpractice is Wickline v. State.[25] In that case, the plaintiff, Lois Wickline, was diagnosed with Leviche's syndrome, a vascular condition. Her physician recommended surgery, which was preapproved along with 10 days of postoperative inpatient care by her state-funded health plan, Medi-Cal. After the surgery and 9 days of care, Ms. Wickline's physician determined that she required an additional 8 days of hospital care before being discharged. He sought approval from Medi-Cal, which on the basis of its consultant's recommendation approved only a 4-day extension. The treating physician did not dispute Medi-Cal's determination, and Ms. Wickline was discharged after the extra 4 days had elapsed. Shortly after returning home, Ms. Wickline began to show signs of infection and loss of circulation in her leg. She returned to the hospital (via the emergency room) 9 days after discharge, and her badly infected leg was amputated above the knee.

Wickline brought suit against Medi-Cal alleging that the consultant's negligence in approving only a 4-day discharge extension caused her to be discharged prematurely, and that she would not have lost her leg had she been given the full 8 extra days as requested by her physician.[26]

---

24. The damage award was later reduced by the court.
25. 228 Cal. Rptr. 661 (Ct. App. 1986).
26. Interestingly, the plaintiff did not sue her physician. From a procedural standpoint, the plaintiff needed to allege that the doctor's care had been appropriate to establish that the negligent actions of Medi-Cal proximately caused her injuries without any break in the causal chain. Therefore, suing her physician would have been directly counter to her claim against Medi-Cal. *See* M. R. Kohler, When the Whole Exceeds the Sum of Its Parts: Why Existing Utilization Management Practices Don't Measure Up, 53 U. Pitt. L. Rev. 1061, 1073 (1992).

After a $500,000 verdict for Ms. Wickline at trial, the Appeals Court reversed the lower court's decision, ruling that Medi-Cal was not liable for her injuries. In the view of the Appeals Court, the decision to discharge Ms. Wickline after 4 days was not made by Medi-Cal but by her physician.[27] The court did recognize that an MCO's refusal to approve requested medical services could result in serious consequences for a patient and that an MCO could be found liable when medically inappropriate decisions were made on the basis of errors within the MCO system, such as defects in the implementation of effective UR or appeal procedures.[28] In this case, however, the court reasoned that the physician himself made and implemented a decision to discharge the patient independently of the UR reviewers recommendations.[29]

The *Wickline* court, *in dicta*, criticized the actions of the physician, noting that he could have appealed the denial of his request for an 8-day discharge extension within the MCO system.[30] Furthermore, the court noted that no matter what liability may fall on the MCO, the physician ultimately remained liable to his patients.

> [T]he physician who complies without protest with the limitations imposed by a third party payor, when his medical judgment dictates otherwise, cannot avoid his ultimate responsibility for his patient's care. He cannot point to the health care payor as the liability scapegoat when the consequences of his own determined medical services go sour.[31]

Although the Appeals Court recognized that the MCO put pressure on the physician to comply with its approval limitations, in the court's eyes the physician "was not paralyzed . . . nor rendered powerless to act appropriately if other action was required under the circumstances."[32]

Ultimately, two concepts from the *Wickline* decision are of importance for physicians. First, the court made it clear that a physician's duty to patients is unaffected by the financial pressure of an MCO. Second, the opinion suggests that in certain situations, physicians might have an affirmative duty to advocate on behalf of their patients when an MCO or other payor makes a determination that could adversely affect the patient. Unfortunately, the *Wickline* court offered no guidance in defining the extent of this duty, and physicians are left to determine on a case-by-case basis

---

27. *Wickline* at 670.
28. *Id.*
29. *Id.* at 671.
30. *Id.*
31. *Id.*
32. *Id.*

whether they have tried hard enough to get their patients all possible services.

Following *Wickline*, the California Appeals Court had a chance to revisit the issue of MCO cost cutting. In *Wilson v. Blue Cross of Southern California*,[33] the family of a psychiatric patient sued Blue Cross and a UR firm, alleging that the patient committed suicide because the defendants had failed to provide him with sufficient inpatient services. The patient's psychiatrist had recommended 3–4 weeks of inpatient care to treat the patient's drug dependence and depression. Blue Cross, however, approved only an 11-day stay, following the recommendation of the UR firm they had hired.

After 11 days, the patient was released, with the psychiatrist noting in the record, "patient did well in the program, but had to leave early because of pressure from [the UR firm]." Twenty days later, the patient committed suicide.

The trial court, following the *Wickline* decision, granted summary judgment to the defendants. On appeal, the Appeals Court reversed the lower court, ordering the case to proceed to trial.[34] In its ruling, the Appeals Court revisited *Wickline* and limited that decision's effect on MCO liability. It reread *Wickline* as determining that the release of the patient after 4 extra days fell within the standard of care and not as a decision based on the physician's independent medical decision to discharge Wickline.[35] *The Wilson* Court recognized that in practice, a physician's medical decisions can be strongly affected by the MCO, and the key for the court was whether or not the MCO's actions were the cause of the patient's suicide.[36]

As with the *Wickline* decision, the *Wilson* opinion offers little concrete advice for the physician. The Court failed to characterize the duty of the MCO or that of the physician operating within the MCO environment. What the *Wilson* decision does offer is the judicial recognition that MCO policies affect the care provided to patients to such an extent that liability can be imposed on an MCO under certain circumstances.[37] The physician, however, is still left wondering whether MCO liability will have any effect on the physician's duties.

33. 271 Cal. Rptr. 876 (Ct. App. 1990).
34. The defendant UR firm settled with plaintiffs before trial. Blue Cross was ultimately found not liable on the claim of wrongful death, but liable under a breach of contract claim relating to the patient's contact with Blue Cross. The parties then settled prior to an appeal. *See* D. Azevedo, Courts let UR Firms off the Hook—and Leave Doctors On, Medical Economics, Jan. 25, 1993 at 30.
35. *Wilson* at 879.
36. *Id.* at 883.
37. *See also Corcoran v. United HealthCare, Inc.,* 965 F. 2d 1321 (5th Cir.), *cert. denied,* 113 S. Ct. 812 (1993) (stating that utilization review could constitute independent medical decision-making and that UR denials clearly can affect the medical decisions of patients and providers.

Wilson has not yet spawned many "copy cat" cases. One reason for this is that most courts rule that federal legislation regulating pensions effectively preempts the ability of an insured patient to sue if the insurance is part of an employment benefit. A case in point is *Elsesser v. Hospital of the Philadelphia College of Osteopathic Medicine.*[38] In that case, suit was brought against the hospital, certain doctors, and an HMO by representatives of a patient who had suffered cardiac arrest. Before the arrest, her doctor had ordered her to use a Holter monitor but discontinued it after being told by the HMO that it would not pay. The court ruled that the HMO's decision not to pay was a matter of plan coverage governed by federal pension law and that the claims against the HMO were barred. *Elsesser* and similar cases raise the very unpleasant possibility that the physician, after succumbing to MCO pressure, will find that the MCO will escape any liability whatsoever, and the physician alone will be left to answer in court.

As the above decisions illustrate, the judicial system is having a difficult time reconciling modern economics-driven health care with traditional notions of malpractice. To date, courts have clung to the belief that a physician should not consider the economic consequences of medical decision making. At the same time, as the *Wickline* and *Wilson* decisions indicate, courts are beginning to recognize that the systems implemented by MCOs to save money inevitably affect physician practice. Most courts, however, have applied this concept by looking at expanding liability beyond the physicians to the MCO itself or related entities such as UR firms. No court has explicitly stated that a physician's duty is *decreased* because of the MCO's cost-cutting techniques. As a result, physicians remain in an unenviable position, caught between the Scylla of UR and Charybdis of malpractice.

Practical Implications for the Physician

Depending on the cost-control structure imposed by the MCO, it may be vital for the physician to document attempts to intervene on the patient's behalf in the reimbursement system.

If the system is essentially a fee-for-service model and the UR review is retrospective, the malpractice implications are relatively minor, since by definition the service has already been performed by the time cost cutting comes into play. To put it another way, effort expended by the physician in seeking reimbursement cannot affect the quality of past care.[39]

---

38. 802 F. Supp. 1286 (E.D. Penn. 1992).
39. A plaintiff could possibly complain that the physician's prospect of not getting paid affected his clinical decision making. If the MCO has disciplined, expelled, or punished doctors based on retroactive UR findings, this argument would be strengthened.

If, however, the UR is concurrent or prospective, the physician runs a substantial risk of criticism for "giving in" to financial pressure by providing less than adequate medical practice. In this context, the physician needs to document clearly his or her own medical recommendations. Those recommendations should not be changed without a documented *medical* reason. If the care cannot be given because payment will not be made, then the physician should not take it upon himself or herself to adopt and implement this UR decision. The physician should consider presenting the patient (or patient's family, as appropriate) with any economic decision that will have to be made, along with the physician's *medical* recommendation. If there is an appeal possible from the initial UR decision, the physician should offer to support that effort if the patient desires it. The physician should keep a record of the information he or she has provided to the UR decision makers.[40]

Utilization review in a fee-for-service environment provides an opportunity for the physician to take a medical position and force the MCO to countermand it explicitly. In the process, a record is created, and it is relatively easy for the physician to demonstrate to the patient that he or she is "on the patient's side." The risk is that the physician will be perceived by the MCO as a medical gadfly who is sowing dissension among patients and making the MCO "look bad." In fact, some MCOs seek to enforce contractual "gag" rules that prevent physicians from communicating with patients concerning plan coverage. Moreover, the attempt to preserve and foster the patient's sense that the physician is an ally may not necessarily protect the physician from a lawsuit.

By contrast, in a system in which cost control is accomplished by capitation, either at the physician level or the level of the physician's group or network, the incentive to keep costs down has been internalized in the physician. There is not necessarily any interplay between the UR apparatus and the physician during which the physician can take a stand. Indeed, it is one of the enticements to capitation that the physician will not be subject to extensive UR bureaucracy, may save time and effort otherwise spent in the UR process, and may feel more freedom in making medical decisions. One price of this freedom is that the motives of the physician in withholding care may be deeply suspect to the patient. Certainly, if a lawsuit arises over whether additional care should have been provided, a plaintiff's attorney will not hesitate to point out to a jury that the extra care would have meant money out of the physician's pocket; and, because there is unlikely to have been any dialogue with the UR system, it may be

---

40. In at least some states this would not be an appropriate part of the medical record and might have to be maintained as a separate record.

difficult for a capitated physician to rebut completely the inference that he or she acted out of greed.

In practical terms, this may mean that the capitated physician should look for extra medical support for the decisions made. Medical guidelines and protocols, although their use may not be decisive, can provide some of this support. The value of guidelines in validating care choices depends on (among other things) their source, their method of adoption, their acceptance within the medical community, their clarity, and the extent to which their underlying bases are disclosed.[41]

In addition, the inference that money motivated the physician's care may be rebutted by financial information that clearly shows that the care in question would not have "broken the bank." In this respect, the financial health of the physician's practice may become a contested element in the malpractice arena.[42]

So far, there are no clear resolutions to the malpractice issues raised by cost-control measures in managed care. Plaintiffs, physicians, MCOs, and the courts themselves are feeling their way through a maze of legal and ethical problems. It is possible that the opportunities for improved quality of care that managed care offers can be emphasized so that the issues surrounding malpractice will have greatly diminished significance. If so, this is one way out of the maze. Whether the managed care system will make use of this opportunity remains to be seen.

LEGAL IMPLICATIONS OF MANAGED CARE CONTRACT PROVISIONS

In the medical world, before the intensive push toward managed care, a physician's contractual relationships were relatively simple. Doctors contracted with their patients to provide them with medical care and advice in return for fees. The physician also frequently joined the hospital's medical staff to gain admitting privileges. Although many courts have seen this relationship with the hospital as essentially contractual, some state courts have recognized extracontractual obligations that require the hospital to meet standards of fair procedure to protect physicians' rights to obtain or retain staff privileges. With the growth of managed care, physicians inevitably have been drawn into more complex contractual relations with

---

41. *See* C. Havinghurst, Practice Guidelines As Legal Standards Governing Physician Liability, 54 Law & Contemp. Prob. 87 (1991).

42. The inference might also be rebutted by evidence of adequate underutilization controls exerted by the MCO. However, it is unlikely that the results of MCO underutilization analysis would be available or admissible at trial. The existence of such controls, coupled with a track record by the physician and/or statistical data demonstrating that the care choice was consistent with other choices may help to rebut an allegation of self-interest. Although this latter type of data almost certainly could not be used to prove the standard of care, it might well be admissible on the issue of the physician's motive.

MCOs. These contracts frequently compel physicians to enter into further contractual arrangements with third parties to limit costs and attain goals set in the original MCO contracts. Many physicians are not familiar with the process of evaluating and establishing these relationships. Indeed, many physicians, viewing their "real job" to be that of health care provider and not businessperson, simply ignore the process of evaluating or negotiating these contracts.[43] Yet, an understanding of these contracts is essential, since in most circumstances courts will enforce the contracts as written, and the physician's rights rarely extend beyond the four corners of the document.

A Summary of Basic Contract Principles

Courts view contracts as participant-defined sets of legal rights and obligations. The courts look to the intent of the parties in determining the nature and limits of those rights and obligations, and over the course of time, the legal system has adopted a set of principles for discerning and enforcing that intent.[44]

A court will first decide whether a contract has, in fact, been made and is enforceable. The classic contract involves a "meeting of the minds" when a promise is made with respect to the exchange of services, property, or money.[45] There must be an exchange of "consideration," which typically means that something more than a promise must be provided to bind the parties. One formulation is that the promisee must suffer detriment (in the sense that they do or promise to do something they are not legally obligated to do), the detriment must induce the promise, and the promise must induce the detriment.[46] Legal detriment must be bargained for and exchanged for the promise.[47]

Contracts will not be enforced if they are unconscionable or against public policy. Unconscionability implies a serious violation of moral values; for example, an agreement that is so one-sided as to put one party entirely at the mercy of another and in which one party acts to lure the party into the contract may be struck down as unconscionable. The public policy exception involves a societal choice not to enforce certain agreements. In the area of managed care, courts will use one or more of these principles to nullify managed care contracts that involve Medicare fraud[48] or that violate antitrust law.[49]

---

43. It is not unusual to encounter physicians who have not even read their MCO contracts.
44. Corbin on Contracts §538 (West, St. Paul 1960 & 1994 Supp.)
45. *See* H. O. Hunter, Modern Law of Contracts (Warren, Gorham & Lamont Boston 1987).
46. *See,* e.g., *Allegheny College v. Nat'l Chautauqua Cty. Bank,* 246 N.Y. 369 (1927).
47. *See* J. D. Calamari & J. M. Perillo, *Contracts* at 134–135 (2nd Ed. West, St. Paul 1977).
48. *See Polk Cty. v. Peters,* 800 F. Supp. 1451, 1456 (E.D. Tex. 1992).
49. *Cf. Kaiser Alum. & Chem. Sales, Inc. v. Avondale Shipyards, Inc.,* 677 F. 2d 1045, 1058–60 (5th Cir. 1982) (discussing violation of antitrust laws as defense to actions in contract).

Courts will not enforce contracts in which one party has been misled into signing or in which the contract is based on a mutual mistake of fact. If one contracting party misrepresents (even innocently) a fact upon which the other relies in entering the contract, the misled party may be able to avoid the contract.[50]

If there is an enforceable contract, a court will look to the contract's "plain" language to decide what the parties are obligated to do. Generally, if that language can be construed in a way that is internally consistent with other parts of the contract and not ambiguous, courts will enforce it as written. Some exceptions to this rule include cases in which performance of the contract has become impossible because of a truly unforeseen state of affairs,[51] or cases in which a party has not acted fairly and in good faith.[52] The key concept is that the "intent" that courts enforce is usually inferred from the contract itself, not from the subjective beliefs of the parties.[53]

If, on the other hand, the contract language is ambiguous, then a court may attempt to determine what the contract means. To do this, courts frequently look behind the contract to find its meaning, occasionally finding meaning based on the conduct between the parties before and during the performance of the contract, as well as on conventions in the area of commerce in which the two parties are engaged.[54] Similarly, the respective parties' intent as embodied in communications from one to the other will be referenced.[55] Therefore, physicians should consider conducting negotiations in writing to preserve the statements of inducement, purpose, and position that the parties exchanged in reaching a final agreement. Again, what is in a party's "heart-of-hearts" is largely irrelevant; the only significant statements of intent are those that were communicated, were documented, and can be proven in a court of law.

Moreover, a contract will be construed against the party who drafts it.[56] This principle has significance to physicians who are presented by MCOs with "boilerplate" contracts on a take-it-or-leave-it basis. Although such

---

50. However, in many cases, if the "misled" party has in fact made its own investigation of the matter before making the agreement, the contract will stand. *See*, e.g., *McCormick & Co. v. Childers*, 468 F.2d 757 (4th Cir. 1972).

51. Thus, for example, if a PHO requires a physician to admit PHO-covered patients only into the PHO hospital, the contract may be unenforceable if the hospital burns down.

52. Many state courts read a "constructive condition" into contracts that creates a duty for the parties to deal fairly and in good faith with each other. *See* 17A Am. Jur. 2d §380(1991 & 1995 Supp.).

53. This approach is reinforced by the so-called parole evidence rule, which provides that if the document appears to be "integrated" (purports to contain the parties' only effective terms), parole evidence (evidence of circumstances surrounding the contract and its making) will not be considered.

54. *See* Corbin on Contracts §562 (West, St. Paul 1960 & 1994).

55. Williston On Contracts §621 (3rd Ed. 1961 & 1994 Supp.).

56. *Id.* at §601.

contracts have usually been carefully constructed to avoid ambiguity, any ambiguous language generally will be construed against the writer (i.e., the MCO).

In choosing how to write a contract, reliance on the principles of contract interpretation that a court might apply in subsequent litigation is a very risky proposition. It is better to establish a clear written understanding on the key points and so avoid later conflict and disagreement. However, since medical care involves many unforeseeable situations, it is sometimes necessary to provide "loose" terms that give the parties leeway in an uncertain future. Of course, the disadvantage is that such language will be seen as ambiguous, and a court may embark on an interpretive search through the surrounding facts to determine what the parties intended.

Factors to Consider in Evaluating Managed care Contracts

Prior to negotiating a managed care contract, all physicians should have a working knowledge of the major issues and pitfalls.[57] In this regard, physicians may find substantial help from professional medical societies, some of which have useful guides available to their members.[58]

ANTITRUST

As discussed in greater detail below, several laws intended to foster competition limit the manner in which physicians (or groups of physicians) and MCOs can contract with each other.[59] Agreements that may appear to make economic sense to the physician, in fact, may be unlawful, and the illegal nature of the transaction may be counterintuitive. All managed care contracts should therefore be reviewed carefully for antitrust violations.[60]

FRAUD AND ABUSE

Another area of government regulation that can create restrictions on business dealings with MCOs are the fraud and abuse restrictions dis-

---

57. In addition, any physician entering into such a contract would do well to have an informed legal counsel.
58. *See*, e.g., *The Physician and Managed Care,* American Medical Association (Chicago 1993); *Managed Care Contract Review Checklist,* Texas Medical Association; *Physician's Managed Care Manual,* California Medical Association; *Contracts for Anesthesiological Care,* American Society of Anesthesiologists (Park Ridge, Ill. 1994).
59. See "Government Regulation: Antitrust," this chapter.
60. As a practical matter, when a physician is bargaining with an MCO that is not composed of other, potentially competing physicians, the risk of antitrust violations is decreased. Even deals with large institutions such as HMOs and hospitals, however, should be given careful legal screening.

cussed in more detail below.[61] These criminalize many business relationships that are assumed to distort the market for government-reimbursed medical services and equipment.

Since these statutes are extremely broad in scope, the effort is usually made in any contract to qualify under one of several "safe harbors," or exceptions from prosecution. These safe harbors themselves are somewhat vaguely drawn, so that there can be substantial risk in almost any transaction. Moreover, the scope of these statutes is a matter of constant proposed change and/or judicial clarification. What appears legal today may be illegal tomorrow and vice versa. If you are relying on a representation by the MCO that the deal is legal, consider asking for a written opinion, preferably from the MCO's counsel, that assures you of legality and expressly states that you (as opposed to just the MCO) may rely upon it.[62]

MCO RELIABILITY

MCOs may go bankrupt, leaving creditors, including physicians, with claims that are difficult or impossible to collect in full. In the fast-shifting market for health care services, consolidations and competitive showdowns materialize overnight. A physician must accurately gauge the financial soundness of any MCO with which he or she contracts. Many MCOs are regulated and file financial information with government agencies. The physician should obtain all public information and consider requesting further disclosure of the MCO's financial position before entering into any contract.

Closely related to this is information about the MCO's current and historical business practices. Is it a "slow pay"? Does it have a history of denying many provider claims? Is it administratively difficult to deal with? Does it have a history of severing physician contracts as part of a marketing strategy?

ISSUES OF DISCRETION AND CONTROL

Many MCO contracts contain language that gives substantial discretion to one or both of the parties. For example, an MCO may only pay for care that is "necessary" or "appropriate," or a practice-group contract may require a physician to be "reasonably" available. Given the nature of medical care and the types of activities that physicians undertake, use of some

---

61. See "Government Regulation: Fraud and Abuse," this chapter.
62. As a practical matter, such an opinion, especially one that is not heavily conditioned and qualified, will be hard to get. However, if an opinion is simply addressed to the MCO and not to you, you may not be able to make any claim under the lawyer's malpractice policy, should the opinion be in error.

such general terms is almost inevitable. Further definition may be impossible at the time of contracting or not desirable from one or both parties' point of view.

When terms are used that can change meaning depending upon circumstances, the key issue is the procedure that will be used to determine the meaning. Many MCO contracts seek to reserve to the MCO the discretion to define terms as needed. Courts will frequently uphold such reservations of discretion and will not second-guess the deciding party without a clear abuse of discretion.[63]

Thus physicians *must* understand who will make these judgment calls and what procedures will be followed in making them. Some MCOs permit physicians to challenge decisions internally through committees or appeals to administrators. The physician needs to know who will make decisions at the various levels, including whether the decisions will be made by an MD or someone else likely to understand the issue from the physician's point of view. Furthermore, the physician should know if he or she will have an early opportunity to communicate with the decision maker to head off any misunderstanding. If the physician disagrees with the decision, an opportunity to make an appeal is desirable. On one hand, if any appeal process is cumbersome, as it can be with an appeals committee, the process can lose much of its value to a physician whose income may be hanging in the balance. On the other hand, a "quick" appeal may sacrifice the physician's ability to present his or her case carefully and may vest discretion in a single individual who is more apt to act arbitrarily.

These considerations should be balanced in light of the nature of the MCO and the nature of the decision being made. Simple payment decisions for individual services should not require complex appeal machinery; whereas decisions that reflect on global payments or the quality of the physician's care or on the continuation of the contract merit a more elaborate (and more time-consuming) process. Among other things, physicians should look for the ability to present their case to the decision maker, the existence within the MCO contract of guidelines or standards that help to predict an outcome, and the creation of a record of written justification for any "final" decision. If the decision involves criticism of the physician's capabilities, the physician should look for provisions allowing for notice of any charges and an opportunity to review and dispute adverse statements and documents.

The issue of who gets to exercise discretion also has a substantial impact on possible liability for patient care decisions. As discussed above,

---

63. This kind of reservation is especially common in contracts involving personal service to one party's satisfaction. *Williston on Contracts* §675A (3rd Ed., 1961 & 1994 Supp.).

physicians find themselves in a "heads you win, tails I lose" situation in which they are seen as responsible for the quality of care rendered, even if certain financial decisions that impact on that care are out of their control.[64] Yet, the MCOs themselves are also walking a very narrow line. On one hand, they want to control the nature, quality, and quantity of care provided, since this is the heart and soul of cost-efficient care; on the other hand, the more control they exercise over medical decisions, the more likely they are to be sued if something goes wrong.

In many MCO contracts, the MCO tries to solve this problem by making the physician an independent contractor. In most business contexts, an independent contractor is one who approaches a job using his or her own discretion, independently determining how the job will be done.[65] There is a substantial body of case law as to how and when someone will qualify as an independent contractor. In the MCO contract context, this qualification can be important for tax purposes, since physicians may have tax-deferred pension arrangements that are predicated upon their status as independent contractors and not as employees of an MCO. Regardless of any label applied in the contract, the IRS will look at various criteria to determine whether employment actually exists.[66] If the physician is deemed to be an employee by the IRS, the tax consequences for any pension plan that was set up under the assumption that the physician was an independent contractor will be very serious.

If the physician is a bona fide employee of the MCO, there is an extensive body of statutory case law that affords the physician many substantial rights. These rights extend from federal statutes forbidding discriminatory behavior based on race, sex, and disability to legislatively and judicially created legal principles protecting employees against bad faith terminations and retaliation for "whistle-blowing."[67]

Although MCO contracts are usually quite careful to define the physi-

---

64. *See* "Legal Implications of Managed Care Contract Provisions," this chapter.
65. *See* Restatement (Second) Agency, §2 (1958); *Williston on Contracts,* §1012A (3rd Ed. 1961).
66. In the context of other industries, the IRS has used a 20-factor test to determine if an employment relationship is created. *See* Rev. Rul. 87–41, 1987–1 C.B 296. These factors include whether the "employer" hires assistants and provides training, tools, and supplies for the "employee" and whether the "employer" determines when, where, and how work is to be done. However, the IRS recognizes that in the medical context, physicians almost always retain control over medical decision making; and, instead of looking at who controls the physician's medical work, the IRS focuses instead on who controls the physician's business operations. Among other things, the IRS will look at factors such as whether the physician works exclusively for the MCO, whether compensation is related to fees collected, whether the physician gets employee-type benefits, and whether the MCO bears the business expenses related to staffing, office space, insurance, and other expenses. *See* IRS Coursebook on Introduction to the Health Care Industry.
67. These protections have created a body of rapidly growing legal precedent in the area of employment law that cannot be summarized within a single chapter. However, physicians should be aware that when an employment relationship is created, this body of law can be invoked to restrict the employer's freedom to do as it pleases.

cian as an independent contractor,[68] they frequently require physicians or physician groups to "direct," "instruct," or "supervise" the work of nurses and technicians, even though these people are employed by the MCO and not the physicians. This raises the possibility that a physician will be liable for any mistakes these nonphysicians may make.

In settings such as hospitals, courts have been split over whether physicians, who have traditionally had the power to direct hospital employees, are liable for the employees' negligence. One string of cases permits doctors to rely on the independent judgment of such workers about routine matters without sharing liability for their acts.[69] Other cases essentially look to the physician as responsible for those under his or her "command."[70] When an MCO/physician contract expressly recognizes this command function, the risk of physician liability is increased, since legal responsibility tends to follow legal control.[71]

One way to address this problem is to have the physician receive an indemnification from the MCO.[72] Of course, the value of such indemnification depends upon the financial resources of the MCO. To ensure that resources are available to pay claims, the MCO may obtain insurance. A physician who is going to rely on the MCO's insurance policy should make sure that the policy is in an amount that will realistically cover liability in today's malpractice environment. The physician should also make sure that he or she is named as an insurance beneficiary or covered person if possible.

PHYSICIAN ADMINISTRATIVE FUNCTIONS

Often, MCO contract provisions require physicians to perform administrative tasks for the MCO. For example, a physician might have to participate in budgeting, credentialing, or scheduling or in recruitment and evaluation of physicians or nonphysician MCO employees.

Such provisions raise questions of adequate compensation and the necessity for limiting burdensome tasks. Physicians must know what kind

---

68. Exceptions to this include staff model HMOs and practice groups that employ physicians.
69. Prosser & Keeton on Torts, *supra* note 6, at 204, n. 10.
70. *Id.* at p. 189, n. 57 & p. 204, n. 15.
71. An issue closely related to the physician's control of the MCO's employees for purposes of tort liability is whether those employees become employees of the physician for tax purposes. Even when an employee receives his or her salary from another entity, it is possible to "lease" employees and be held responsible for certain obligations, such as employee pension requirements. This is a somewhat arcane area of tax law; but, if MCO employees are going to spend much of the time working for the physician, the physician should demand and receive adequate legal assurance that he or she will not be considered an employer.
72. MCOs commonly require physicians to indemnify them from liability caused by physician acts and omissions. There is no reason why a reciprocal indemnity shouldn't be given to physicians for liability caused by the acts and omission of the MCO and its employees.

of limit can be placed on such activities. Otherwise, the physician or physician group may find that a fixed contract fee calculated on care given is insufficient to compensate for the combined care and administrative duties required under the contract. Without a limit on administrative burdens, the MCO may be tempted to cut its own administrative overhead by shuffling paperwork onto the physician's desk.

Liability issues also arise when physicians are required to perform administrative duties. One common activity frequently required of physicians by MCOs is participation in the system's peer review process. Although federal and state statutes generally provide protection for peer review activities,[73] there are some MCO environments in which such statutes are inapplicable.[74] In addition, very few statutes provide "airtight" protection from lawsuits.[75] Physicians, therefore, should look for indemnification from the MCO for liabilities arising out of these administrative duties and should consider requesting insurance coverage with the physician as named insured to any liability that does arise.

MCO DUTIES

Although physician/MCO contracts usually attempt to specify the duties or functions that the physician must perform, they frequently do not say much about the MCO's reciprocal obligations, other than to pay compensation.[76]

Nevertheless, when the parties are made to focus on the issue, it usually becomes apparent that the MCO has obligations that are every bit as essential to the successful function of the contract as those of the physician, and these should be explicitly listed. For example, depending on the circumstances, the MCO may have to provide facilities, access, equipment, and nonphysician support for the physicians to do their job. In addition, it may be part of the MCO's "job" to bargain on behalf of physician members with other MCOs or to promote the use of physician services to the public. In almost every case, it is in the physician's interests to specify these MCO obligations and, if possible, to establish contractual benchmarks for proper performance. If these cannot be specified, general reference to obligations (e.g., to provide "reasonable" or "adequate" facilities),

---

73. The federal statute is 42 U.S.C. §§11101–11151 also known as the Health Care Quality Improvement Act of 1986 (HCQIA). All 50 states have enacted peer-review immunity laws. *See Note, Patrick v. Burget: The Future of Hospital Peer Review Committees in the Antitrust Arena,* 39 DePaul L. Rev. 881, 890–91 n. 69 (1990).

74. For example, the HCQIA does not cover PPOs.

75. P. L. Scibetta, *Note: Restructuring Hospital-Physician Relations: Patient Care Quality Depends on the Health of Hospital Peer Review,* 51 U. Pitt L. Rev. 1025, 1033 (1990).

76. This is understandable since most contracts are drafted in the first instance by the MCO or its counsel.

even though vague, can give the physician a basis on which to attempt to correct the MCO's behavior if it is found wanting.

A contact is of necessity a two-way street. Every physician should ask "what will you be doing for me?" and should require that the answer be part of any written agreement.

CREDENTIALING AND TERMINATION

In the traditional physician/hospital relationship, the physician's rights to join and stay on the staff are governed by a series of procedural safeguards based on both federal and state law. Under the federal Health Care Quality Improvement Act of 1986, the hospital's credentialing/peer review system must be fair in order for hospitals to qualify for certain immunities. The statute lists certain basic procedural safeguards that fulfill this fairness requirement, such as

Notice of the charges against a physician; the opportunity for a hearing; the place, time and date of the hearing; and the identity of witnesses
A disinterested decision maker
The right to representation
The creation of a record
The right to cross-examine and call witnesses
A written decision including a statement of the basis for the decision

When hospitals are state run or when the hospital's relation with the state is so closely symbiotic as to make the state a joint participant in hospital decisions, constitutional due process requirements mandate that similar procedures be followed.[77] Courts in a number of states have also required privately run hospitals to afford staff physicians the rudiments of due process, based upon an argument that because hospitals control access to a type of care and thus a segment of the care market, they cannot bar physicians from entry without following a fundamentally fair process.[78] In other states, the physician/hospital relationship is seen as contractual, with the physician getting only those rights stated in staff bylaws.[79] By convention or tradition, the bylaws in those states frequently

---

77. *See, e.g., Woodbury v. McKinnon*, 447 F. 2d 839 (5th Cir. 1971); *Shaw v. Hospital Auth. of Cobb Cty.*, 507 F. 2d 625 (5th Cir. 1975), *aff'd on reh.*, 614 F. 2d 946 (5th Cir. 1980). However, where a doctor is employed by a hospital on an "at will" basis, the termination of his or her employment need not involve procedural due process. *See Engelstad v. Virginia Mun. Hosp.*, 718 F. 2d 262 (8th Cir. 1983).
78. *See, e.g., Greisman v. Newcomb Hospital*, 40 N.J. 389 (1963); *Applebaum v. Bd. of Dir. of Barton Mem. Hosp.*, 104 Cal. App. 3d 648, 163 Cal. Rptr. 831 (1980); *Siquera v. Northwestern Hosp.*, 87 Ill. Dec. 415, 477 N.E. 2d (Ill. 1985).
79. *See, e.g., Lewisburg Comm. Hosp. v. Algredson*, 805 S.W. 2d 756 (Tenn. 1991); *Saint Louis v. Baystate Med. Center*, 30 Mass. App. Ct. 393, 568 N.E. 2d 1181 (1991); *Bartley v. Eastern Maine Med. Center*, 617 A. 2d 1020 (Me. 1992).

provide very substantial procedural protections. The Joint Commission on the Accreditation of Health Organizations (JCAHO) has in the past proposed certain similar procedural safeguards, and various states have incorporated these into their law.

Unfortunately, in managed care, the physician's rights against an MCO are largely defined by contact, and procedural protections may only exist if they are set forth in the contract.[80] In the current economic climate, MCOs are not willing to burden themselves with wholesale grants of complex procedural rights. Nevertheless, at least one case has suggested that physicians may enjoy inherent, noncontractual, due process rights with MCOs.

In *Delta Dental Plan of Cal. v. Banasky,*[81] two dentists had signed up with Delta and agreed to be bound by its rules. The dentists were to provide a list of usual fees, which, if accepted by Delta, would be used to make reimbursement. Upon learning that the dentists were receiving lesser reimbursement from another MCO, Delta reduced its own fee level retroactively. The court relied on California legal precedent in hospital cases to find that the dentists had a right to fair procedure to protect them from exclusion from, or sanctions by, organizations that control important economic interests. The court concluded that in light of this procedural safeguard, the dentists had to challenge the decision first through Delta's own internal appeal process.

Delta Dental is a double-edged sword. It initially recognizes a right to fair process, but relegates the provider to follow the process afforded by the MCO. Its frank application of state administrative procedure statutes to MCO decision making is far beyond any protection known to this chapter's authors to be provided to MCO physicians in any other state.

It remains to be seen whether other courts will apply the same reasoning to MCOs. Certainly, where the MCO effectively controls access by a physician to certain modalities of care, a similar analysis could be applied. In *Delta Dental,* the analysis was tied to MCO control over access to the patients themselves. In states that have imposed inherent (noncontractual) due process standards on hospitals, this theory appears to have substantial force.

As a practical matter, if an MCO contract lacks procedural protections, physicians cannot rely on hospital bylaws to protect their access to staff privileges. Since more and more commonly, access to hospital departments is controlled by MCO affiliation and/or by exclusive contracting, the MCO contract, not the hospital bylaws, can become the determinant of hospital staff participation. Thus, when a hospital department is

---

80. Even in a hospital context, if practice is governed by an exclusive contract, bylaw procedures may be no protection where hospital access is terminated under the contract. *See Dutta v. St. Francis Reg. Med. Center,* 254 Kan 690, 897 P.2d 1057(1994); *Hutton v. Memorial Hosp.,* 824 P. 2d 61 (Col App. 1991).
81. 27 Cal. App. 4th 1598, 33 Cal. Rptr. 2d 381 (1994).

"closed"[82] by an exclusive contract with an MCO, a physician's loss or failure to get an MCO contract or membership may mean that no privileges with the hospital are available.[83] MCO contracts frequently provide that physicians who leave (or are forced out) of the MCO relationship will be deemed to have "resigned" privileges at relevant hospitals and facilities. Such provisions have been upheld by some courts,[84] and physicians must be sure they fully understand the consequences of termination of an MCO contract.[85]

ECONOMIC CREDENTIALING AND DESELECTION

The physician community has raised a furor over "economic credentialing"—the determination of physician participation in MCOs on the basis of nonmedical, primarily financial criteria.[86] The MCO can make financial decisions about a physician at many different points in the relationship, including the formation of the contract, the renewal of the contract, and utilization review. MCOs are increasingly reserving the right to "audit" physicians office practices, including their financial soundness and business practices. Without any current legislation or regulations, courts have yet to strike down the application of economic criteria as long as use of the economic factor is disclosed in MCO contracts either explicitly or via a general right to terminate a contract "without cause." In fact, some courts are quick to recognize and support even the most tenuous connections between "economic" decisions and the quality care justifications offered by MCOs.[87]

Many physicians' organizations have condemned economic credentialing in official statements.[88] Moreover, several states have adopted "any

---

82. Courts have allowed hospitals to "close" departments based on arguments relating to improved patient care. *See, e.g., Redding v. St. Francis Medical Center,* 255 Cal. Rptr. 806 (Cal. Ct. App. 1989); *Bellam v. Clayton Cty. Hosp. Auth.,* 758 F. Supp. 1488 (N.,D.Ga. 1990). However, attempts to close staffs that are seen as pretexts to consolidate or carry forward the economic position of existing staff participant have been overturned. *See, e.g., Desai v. St. Barnabas Med. Center,* 510 A.2d 662 (N.J. 1986) (closure of staff overturned where exceptions to closure had already been made to replenish existing practice groups).
83. *See Dutta v. St. Francis Reg. Med. Center,* 254 Kan. 690, 867 P. 2d 1057 (1994).
84. *Id.*
85. The right to terminate on short notice and without cause, although it may hurt the physicians, can be a cloud with a silver lining if it is mutual. If the physician is unhappy with the MCO and the contract can be terminated quickly, the physician has an opportunity to vote with his or her feet. However, this may be small consolation for the physician who is summarily terminated.
86. See J. J. Blum, Physician Economic Credentialing—A New Factor in Credentialling, Medial Staff Coun., Winter 1991 at 25–30; H. L. Lang, Economic Credentialling—Why it Must be Stopped, Medical Staff Coun., Spring 1991 at 19–25.
87. *See* M. A. Kadzielski and M. B. Reynolds, Economic Issues and Credentialling Decisions: The Controversy Continues, Health Care Law Newsletter, Vol. 8, No. 3 March 1993 pp. 12–16. A distinction must be drawn between situations that involve antitrust violations and those involving economic credentialing. If credentialing decisions, whether economic or medical, are seen as an attempt by competitors to restrict competitions, the action will be invalid under relevant antitrust law. See "Government Regulation: Antitrust," this chapter. In contrast, if the MCO is a legitimate and integrated business entity, its decisions to limit providers to those who are cost efficient may well be seen by courts as procompetitive and beneficial for the consumer.

willing provider" laws or "patients rights" laws, some of which prevent certain types of MCOs from "deselecting" providers or from refusing to deal with them at their whim.[89] These statutes generally require MCOs to deal with physicians who are willing to abide by MCO requirements related to quality and procedure. Although these statutes may not address economic credentialing directly, they attempt to tilt the balance of power back to providers. Some of these statutes may effectively prevent the creation of closed-panel HMOs, although the legislation is relatively new and its full effect is yet to be seen.

Unfortunately, since MCOs exist to control the cost of medical service, the pressures for the contractual restriction of physician participants and the economic pressure on the MCOs to restrict membership remain acute. MCOs have every incentive to find ways to restrict and control physician activity in ways that are not explicitly forbidden. Thus, an MCO that cannot limit its physician membership by profile of economic "performance" may develop more stringent "quality" criteria that may have the same ultimate effect ("hyperquality" standards). For example, a quality argument may be made that "excessive" patient lengths of stay are a marker of poor quality because the incidence of iatrogenic illness in hospitals is undeniably quite high. A physician with longer than average lengths of stay might thus be deselected on "quality" grounds. Since this type of economic decision may masquerade as merely very tough quality review, which sounds as if it is in the public interest, physicians who are targets may face uphill legal battles in the courts.

From the standpoint of the physician's legal status, it is much less desirable to be subjected to hyperquality credentialing than it is to be subjected to economic credentialing. Under the HCQIA, quality-based credentialing decisions must be reported to the National Practitioners' Data Bank and to local licensing authorities. These reports are in turn accessible to hospitals, HMOs, and other credentialing institutions. Although a physician who is decredentialed for economic reasons may also end up with unflattering data entries, the physician who is decredentialed for purportedly quality-based reasons stands to have access to other staff positions effectively curtailed.[90]

---

88. *See,* e.g., California Medical Association and California Association of Hospitals and Health Systems, Joint Statement on Economic Credentialling and Exclusive Contracting.

89. About two dozen states currently have such statutes. *See* BNA Health Care Daily, Dec. 2, 1994. These statutes vary greatly in the coverage. In 11 states, the statutes only protect pharmacists.

90. If no antitrust violation is involved, the rule is almost universal that initial refusal to credential a physician based even superficially on quality criteria will be upheld.

COMPENSATION

When contracting with an MCO, a physician must understand the manner in which compensation will be calculated. General formulae, which in the abstract sound fair, may in practice give rise to bitter disputes or actually violate various legal requirements. The physician should not trust that the acceptance of a formula by other physicians, even partners in a group practice, means that the formula will operate rationally or fairly or that it conforms to applicable law.

Compensation systems vary along a spectrum. At one end is salaried employment; at the other is complete capitation, with arrangements from the sharing of group or departmental income to fee-for-service lying in between. As one moves away from salary along the spectrum, financial risk and uncertainty increase for the physician. When at the riskiest end of the spectrum (capitation plans), physicians should look for "stop loss" contract provisions, which provide for additional MCO subsidy when care costs exceed certain limits and which prevent capitated physicians from being financially ruined by catastrophic or anomalous medical problems among their patients.

At the more secure end of the spectrum—employment for salary—fringe benefits become more important, potentially constituting a substantial part of the total compensation package. Physicians should bargain for defined vacation policies, pension benefits, insurance, reimbursements for education expenses, and the opportunity for bonuses. It is also usually in the employee's interest to have clear criteria for salary raises (or reductions). If these are not carefully defined, the employer will be deemed able under the law in most jurisdictions to make or withhold raises "at will" and to reduce salary under the same conditions that would merit firing or laying off the employee.

In cases in which the physician is not actually employed, physicians should be aware that the "real" value of compensation may depend on factors apart from dollars and cents. These include

Provisions specifying who bears the financial risk if the patient or the physician leaves the managed care plan in circumstances under which the physician cannot withdraw from the physician:patient relationship

Provisions specifying the circumstances under which the MCO can require the physician to provide charity or reduced-price services (especially relevant if the MCO has a hospital component)

In cases in which compensation is related to physician or MCO performance, the nature of any mechanism to verify performance; if there is an audit procedure, the physician needs to know who will do the audit and how available the information will be to the physician or to others

In cases in which there is a fee-for-service relationship, the extent to which the physician must accept MCO payment as payment in full, and, the existence, conditions, and amount of any reserve or hold-back by the MCO to guard against overutilization; also important are clear criteria for payment to the physician and clear criteria for overutilization

In cases in which an MCO pays on the basis of a schedule or value guide, the frequency with which the schedule gets updated, the index used for updating, and the nature of provisions for payment for procedures not on the list

Contractual provisions that protect the physician against late processing or payment by the MCO

Requirements that the physician treat all patients who come to the physician as part of the MCO system and the procedure by which a physician can limit the size of (or close) his or her practice

MEDICAL NECESSITY

At the intersection of compensation, discretion, and control are issues of medical necessity. To the extent that an MCO undertakes to pay for care that is medically necessary in a fee-for-service model, the standards it applies and the procedures it follows directly affect compensation.

In an effort to attract patients, MCOs that enroll members frequently seek to keep benefits simple. Rather than promulgating a complex list of procedures and conditions that qualify for payments, MCOs frequently undertake only to pay for care that is "medically necessary." Obviously, what the phrase gains in simplicity, it loses in specificity, and MCOs sometimes provide additional definitions in an attempt to narrow the field of acceptable care.

Defining "medically necessary" can make a major financial difference to the MCO. Because of the MCO's legal sophistication and financial muscle and because the MCO chooses the definition, traditional insurance law dictates that ambiguity in coverage is construed in favor of the policyholder, i.e., the patient.[91] Consistent with this standard, a vague definition of medical necessity in the patient's policy will result in liberal rulings by courts in favor of coverage.[92] This carries with it relative freedom for the physician making care recommendations.

---

91. *See* M. Rhodes, Couch Cyclopedia of Insurance Law, §15:74 (Rev. Ed. 1984 & 1995 Supp.)

92. *See Bradley v. Empire Blue Cross & Blue Shield*, 562 N.Y.S. 2d 908 (N.Y. Sup. Ct. 1990); *see also* M. Hall & G. Anderson, Health Insurers' Assessment of Medical Necessity, 140 U. Penn. L. Rev. 1637 (1992); *Van-Vactor v. Blue Cross Ass'n*, 365 N.E.2d 638 (Ill. Ct. App. 1977).

When contracting with an MCO, it is important to know not only the MCO's stated policy but also its procedure for resolving medical necessity issues and its track record for decision making. A number of court cases have addressed the soundness of MCO coverage decisions. For example, failure to interview the physician prior to denial of payment for a procedure[93] and failure to review the entire record prior to such denial[94] have been interpreted as defects in the denial process. In fact, in California, if the MCO wishes to apply a necessity standard different from the community's standards, it must so notify its policyholders.[95]

GOVERNMENT REGULATION: FRAUD AND ABUSE

Managed care organizations seeking to exert influence over a physician's economic and medical care decisions often seek to align the physician's financial interest with their own. This alignment is part of the "integration" of the health care system and typically involves a series of interlocking steps. The alignment between the MCO's and the physician's interests is usually accomplished through a number of financial arrangements by which the physician is presented with a series of financial incentives and restrictions that will, if followed, increase the physician's income, save money for the MCO, and/or attract enrollees to the MCO. In other instances, the purchase of a physician's practice might be coupled with an employment contract into a fully integrated health system. In a system that is less than fully integrated, the payors at the top of the pyramid—the government in the case of Medicare and Medicaid and private payors in other instances—are very aware that the incentives and restrictions they are imposing may encourage physicians to try to "game the system" and cash in on certain incentives to the disadvantage of the patient or the ultimate payor.[96]

As managed care systems have expanded and the cost of medical care has grown, the state and federal legislatures have become increasingly suspicious that a substantial part of the cost increase has been caused by "overutilization" of services, false reporting, or intentional inflation. These legislatures have passed a number of statutes that make false claims as well as various types of financial relationships illegal.[97] In essence, the

---

93. *See McLaughlin v. Connecticut Gen. Life Ins. Co.*, 565 F. Supp. 434 (N.D. Cal. 1983). *But see Jett v. Blue Cross and Blue Shield of Alabama*, 890 F.2d 1137 (11th Cir. 1989).
94. *See Aetna Life Ins. Co. v. Lavoie*, 505 So. 2d 1050, 1052–53 (Ala. 1987); *Hughes v. Blue Cross of Northern Cal*, 263 Cal. Rptr. 850, 857, 215 Cal. App. 3rd 832 (1989), *cert. dism.*, 110 S. Ct. 2200 (1990).
95. *See Hughes, supra*, note 94.
96. *See* H. E. Morreim, Gaming the System: Dodging the Rules, Ruling the Dodgers, Archives of Internal Medicine, 151:443(5)(1991)
97. In addition, the Department of Health & Human Services and the FBI have recently stepped up efforts to root out fraud from federal health programs. *See* R. Pear, Ruling by Court Sets Back Prosecutions in a Test Case on Medicaid and Medicare Referrals, New York Times, April 11, 1995 at A18.

resulting antifraud legislation is another tool for the management of care, since it affects care decisions and the economics of providing care. It is a very blunt form of management, with extreme negative incentives for the physician in the form of criminal liability and civil fines.

The antifraud statutes are written broadly and proscribe many business dealings in the medical care area that in any other context would be usual practice. Moreover, although these laws were established to cover services reimbursed in publicly funded programs—Medicare and Medicaid—in some instances they have been explicitly extended to all third-party reimbursed costs.[98] Since physicians in a managed care market are being called upon to be business people, they must have a grasp of these antifraud restrictions. Some otherwise innocent-appearing business relationships can lead to tremendous liability and perhaps even destroy the physician's practice.

When entering into a deal with a larger business entity, many physicians are tempted to believe that the entity's own counsel has checked all the legal issues. This can be very dangerous. Hospitals, physician groups, and health care corporations have all been hit with antifraud liability, despite access to the "best" legal advice. Moreover, legal opinions given to entities in many instances only serve the purposes and agendas of those entities. In fact, in many cases, courts will not recognize a right to malpractice recovery for someone who is not the actual client of the opining attorney, in the event the opinion is wrong.[99]

To know when and how to seek advice, the physician must have a general sense of the law involved. Fraud and abuse prohibitions fall into three major categories: antikickback laws, restrictions on referrals, and laws against false claims.

As of the time this chapter is going to press, there is a federal legislative initiative for Medicare reform that would ease many federal restrictions in this area. The changes for enactment of at least portions of this initiative appear to be high, but the precise nature of the overall resulting reform is still in doubt.

Among other things, elements of the currently proposed reform include (a) provisions in H.R. 2425 requiring prosecutors of Medicare false claims violations to prove providers knew they were submitting false claims and requiring prosecutors of Medicare kickback claims to prove that any kickback was a "significant" purpose of the alleged illegal arrangement; (b) legislation that would require HHS to provide advisory opinions to guide providers as to what constitutes medicare fraud; (c) legislation allowing antikickback law exceptions where discounts, cost sharing, and other induce-

---

98. As a practical matter, the effect of prohibiting behavior in the context of Medicare and Medicaid alone is to prohibit that behavior in all contexts, since physicians often don't know if bills for medical expenses will be submitted to the government for reimbursement.
99. To put it simply, there is no substitute for the physician obtaining his or her own independent advice.

ments to physicians are offered in a managed care context to reduce overall medical costs; and *(d)* provisions in H.R. 2390 allowing doctors to self-refer for ancillary services in a much wider range of circumstances.

The reader is therefore cautioned to check carefully concerning current law and to apply the following section only in light of any Medicare reform legislation ultimately adopted.

Federal Antikickback Legislation

Under 42 U.S.C. §1320a-7b(b), Congress has prohibited transactions in which value is given in return for someone making a transaction that is payable under Medicare or Medicaid. To incur liability under the statute, the violator must

> Knowingly or willfully solicit, receive, offer, or pay remuneration to induce or in return for *(a)* referral of any individual for, or *(b)* purchase, lease, order, or arrangement for any item or service payable under Medicare or Medicaid.

The penalties for violation range from disqualification from participating in the reimbursement programs to fines up to $25,000 and 5 years in prison. The statute also includes civil penalties.[100]

The statute appears deceptively simple and seems to involve mainly the easy-to-avoid situation of bribery. However, the statutory language covers a number of situations that are unexpected and, in fact, criminalizes many common transactions. Overall, there are relatively few reported cases, and courts in different judicial districts are continuing to "define" this area. Aspects of the statute as interpreted by the courts thus far include the following:

1. The violator must have actual knowledge that his or her offering or paying of reimbursement is unlawful.[101] However, as with any criminal statute that requires intent, state of mind can be inferred from your actions.[102] In effect, if circumstances make it look like you knew the act was unlawful, your own testimony about your subjective state of mind may be little help.
2. You may be found responsible for a violation that is committed by your agent, even if that agent is violating your express polices, as long as the agent is acting generally within the scope of his employment.[101]
3. The intent to commit an illegal act does not have to be your only, or

100. Violations of the statute are prosecuted by the United States Attorney and, with respect to civil penalties, by the Department of Health and Human Services' Office of the Inspector General.
101. *Hanlester Network v. Shalala,* 51 F. 3d 1390, 1400 (9th Cir. 1995).
102. *See* W. R. LaFare and A. W. Scott, Jr., Handbook on Clinical Law, 202–03 (1972).

even the main, purpose. It need only be *one* purpose (*U.S. v. Greber*).[103]
Put another way, only if a payment is wholly attributable to the bona
fide delivery of goods and services can a defendant be sure of avoiding
a finding of intent (*U.S. v. Kats*).[104]

4. Even giving a person the *opportunity* to earn money in a legitimate job
   can be an illegal inducement (*U.S. v. Bay State Ambulance and Hospital
   Rental Service, Inc.*).[105]

5. The government does not have to show that anyone was overpaid or
   suffered financial harm as long as it can show an intent to induce utilization.[105] Mere solicitation or inducement is enough, no actual money
   or value need change hands.[101]

6. As it is defined by the courts, inducement is the *intent* to influence the
   reason or judgment of another; that reason or judgment need not actually be influenced.[101]

Approximately 20 states have laws that resemble the above federal
statute.[106] Salient differences in some states include the lack of a requirement
that the government prove a knowing and willful violation[107] and the application of antikickback laws to privately paid (nongovernmental) services.[108]

The Extended Reach of the Federal Law

Although simple in its form, the federal antikickback law is extensive
in its reach. A physician in a managed care environment will surely encounter enormous economic pressure to enter into forbidden transactions;
knowing which are legal can be especially difficult because most of these
transactions do not involve overt bribery.

The Office of the Inspector General (OIG) has issued a series of "Fraud
Alerts," which help one understand how the government likely will view
certain transactions. These alerts have included statements on joint ventures, waiver of medicare deductibles and copayments, hospital incentives, drug marketing, and clinical laboratory services. Although the alerts
do not have the force of law, they do give valuable guidance to physicians
on how the statute may be applied.

For example, a physician who performs an examination for a fee of $100
would usually expect a Medicare claim for $80 (80% of $100), with the patient paying a $20 copayment. In the economic scramble to attract patients

---

103. 760 F.2d 68, 72 (3rd Cir.), *cert. denied* 474 U.S. 988 (1985).
104. 871 F.2d 105–108 (9th Cir. 1989).
105. 874 F.2d 20–29 (1st Cir. 1989).
106. *See*, e.g., Mass. Gen. Laws c. 118E, §41; West's Fla. Stat. Ann. §409.920; Md. Code art. 27 §230B(5);
Miss. Code §43–13-207; N.M. Stat. AM. §30–44-7; Ill. S.H.A. Ch. 23 §0630: 4D-17.
107. *See* e.g., Mass. c. 118E, § 41; *Cf.* West's Fla. Stat. Am. §409.920(3) (creates an inference that one who
signs a false claim knows it to be false).
108. *See*, e.g., Mass. Gen. Laws, c. 175H, §3.

in the managed care environment, that physician might want to overlook anything but the most token effort to collect the copayment. Under this scenario, the Fraud Alerts warn that federal prosecutors could charge the physician with fraud. Prosecutors would argue that by overlooking the copayment, the physician is actually lowering his or her real charge to $80 and thus should only be charging Medicare $64 (80% of $80). Furthermore, the physician could be viewed as offering remuneration to the patient in the form of waiver of the copayment, thus inducing the patient to purchase Medicare-reimbursed services from him.

The OIG also gives the example of a laboratory that wants to keep a physician's business but is not approved for payment by the managed care plan that covers some of the physician's patients. Under the statute, the laboratory cannot offer to handle the physician's managed care work for free in order to continue to receive other referrals from the physician. The OIG takes the position that this is tantamount to offering a bribe and that the laboratory and any physician who accepts the deal may be guilty of criminal conduct.

Since the statute also proscribes receipt of remuneration, the physician who is at the receiving end of a forbidden transaction is also subject to prosecution. For example, consider a pharmaceutical company that recruits a physician to participate in a drug evaluation program and pays the physician on a per capita basis for keeping a relatively simple record of patients receiving the drug. If the record takes only seconds to fill out and the compensation is anything more than token, there is a real danger that it will be seen as a bribe, and if any of the patients involved are Medicare patients, a criminal violation may exist.[109]

In its search for fraud, the OIG will carefully scrutinize any managed care joint venture or business cooperation agreements. The criteria it will apply include

Whether physicians stand to gain by making referrals
Whether referrals are tracked or encouraged
Whether participation or investment in the venture is conditional on the physician continuing to work in the business generating referrals
Whether a venture participant is already engaged in the venture's business (such as a clinical laboratory that sets up a "joint venture" laboratory in the physician's office but does most of the testing at its central facility)
Who actually owns capital equipment and who actually performs the venture's business functions such as billing and delivery

---

109. Obviously, this type of analysis can be pushed to extremes. For example, it can be argued that the medical information received by a physician from a drug detailer is worth money and is therefore remuneration. Since such information is avowedly given to induce the physician to prescribe a specific drug, this can be a kickback. Although neither the Fraud Alerts nor the courts have gone to this extreme, the incredible breadth of the federal statute and its potential collision with traditional medical business practices is apparent from the example.

Whether the physicians' investment is "disproportionately small" to the returns received

Whether physicians can borrow their investment from another venturer or an affiliated entity

Of special concern in the managed care area are hospital incentives provided to encourage physicians to admit patients. In their efforts to recruit and retain physicians, hospitals sometimes offer a series of benefits. These benefits are illegal if they, in effect, reward physicians for referrals. The OIG will look at a number of criteria including

Whether the physician receives something that depends upon volume of admissions

Whether office space, equipment, training, or services are provided by the hospital free or at significant discount

Whether the physician received an income floor or guarantee

Whether any loans are below market or subject to forgiveness by the hospital

Whether travel, conference, and continuing education expenses are paid

Whether the physician receives below-cost health insurance

Whether the physician receives pay for nominal or even phantom administrative services or consultation duties

These Fraud Alert guidelines are not exclusive. The OIG has been careful to state in each that there may be other factors considered and that the matters covered by the alerts are not exhaustive.

Antikickback Safe Harbors

Because of the tremendous breadth of the federal antikickback law, the federal government has defined a number of safe harbors. Failure to comply with the safe harbors does not necessarily mean that the activity is illegal; however, the legality of activities outside the safe harbors cannot be assured. More than 20 safe harbors have been adopted or currently are proposed.[110] Despite their number, the safe harbors are extremely narrow. Below are those safe harbors applicable to managed care situations and the basic requirements necessary to qualify under each.[111]

CERTAIN INVESTMENT INTERESTS IN SMALL VENTURES

, To qualify under this safe harbor, no more than 40% of the interest in the venture can be held by investors capable of making referrals. The terms can-

---

110. The proposed ones *do not* have the force of law and cannot be relied upon. Also, the federal safe harbors do not necessarily protect the physician from liability under relevant state laws.
111. Additional safe harbors exist with respect to certain warranties from manufacturers, discounts on sales of items, waivers of coinsurance and deductibles, and payments to referral services.

not be related to the volume of business generated from the referrer and must be the same as those offered to nonreferrers. The venture's goods and services cannot be sold preferentially to investors. No more than 40% of the venture's gross revenue can come from business generated by investors. The investors cannot borrow any portion of the invested money from the venture and investment return must be proportional to capital invested.

CERTAIN SPACE AND EQUIPMENT RENTALS AND SERVICE AND MANAGEMENT CONTRACTS

The agreement must be in writing, must specify what is leased or provided, must specify the schedule for service or the use granted, must be for 1 year or more, and must set forth in advance the fee consistent with fair market value and not based on referrals or business generated between the parties. In the case of a service contract, the service provided cannot be the promotion of a business arrangement or any activity that violates law.

CERTAIN SALES OF PHYSICIANS' PRACTICES

The period from the first agreement regarding the sale to the date of the sale itself must be 1 year or less. The selling physician cannot make referrals to the purchaser beyond 1 year after that first agreement, and the seller cannot be in a professional position to make referrals after that year. This safe harbor apparently does not protect sales to nonphysicians such as hospitals.

EMPLOYEES

Payments by an employer to a bona fide employee are protected. "Employee" for these purposes is defined under the Internal Revenue Code.[112]

CERTAIN GROUP PURCHASING ORGANIZATIONS

The GPO must have a written agreement with each participant, specifying payment by vendors of 3% or less of the price of goods or services (or specifying the maximum amount the GPO will be paid), and the GPO must disclose annually to the physician and to the government the amount received from each vendor.

CERTAIN INCREASED COVERAGE, COST SHARING, OR PREMIUM REDUCTIONS OFFERED BY MANAGED CARE PLANS

The benefit must be offered by a health plan that receives a premium and provides insurance or contracts with physicians to provide care. The plan must offer the same benefit to all enrollees and cannot claim the cost

---

112. 26 U.S.C. 3121(d)(2).

of the benefits as bad debt for purposes of calculating reimbursement under Medicare or Medicaid or shift the cost to other payors.

CERTAIN PRICE REDUCTIONS OFFERED TO HEALTH PLANS

Physicians can enter contracts to provide care for a reduced price to managed care plans in exchange for agreements to refer to them. However, the physician cannot claim payment from, or otherwise shift the burden of any reduction onto, Medicare, Medicaid, or any other payers. If the plan gets paid by Medicare or Medicaid on a reasonable-cost basis, the agreement, in addition, must be for 1 year or more, it must specify the care and payment methodology, and the plan must accurately report the amount paid. For plans that are not under contract with the government and are not paid on a cost basis, the agreement must also specify who will file claims for reimbursement and the schedule of physician fees. Furthermore, any requests for Medicare or Medicaid payment must be limited to the fee schedule, and only the party designated in the agreement can submit claims.

Self Referrals

In the late 1980s, Congress became suspicious that physicians who owned interests in ancillary-service providers were unjustifiably referring their patients to those providers to reap higher profits from the service companies. In 1989 Congress enacted 42 U.S.C. §1395 nn (Stark I) to prohibit self-interested referrals to clinical laboratories. In 1993, Congress expanded the Stark prohibitions (Stark II).

The law currently prohibits physicians from making a referral for a covered service to an entity with which the physician or a family member has an ownership or investment interest or a compensation arrangement. The covered services include clinical laboratory services, radiology services (including MRI, CT scans, and ultrasound), inpatient and outpatient hospital services, therapy services in radiation and occupational health, durable medical equipment, and supplies; parenteral and enteral nutrients, equipment, and supplies; prosthetics, orthotics, and prosthetic devices and supplies; outpatient prescription drugs; and home health services.

There are a number of important definitional points. The prohibition relates to both Medicare- and Medicaid-reimbursable services, since states are required to adopt the prohibitions into their Medicaid plans.[113] "Ownership or investment" interest includes any equity, debt, or other relationship in the entity or even the holding company or company holding an interest in the entity providing the services. "Referral" includes not only a physician's request for services or items but also requests for consultation and services ordered or performed by the consulting physician as well as the request by the referring physician for establishment of a plan of care by another physician. A "compensation arrangement" includes direct or indirect remuneration of any kind. "Referral" does not include clinical diagnostic laboratory tests and pathology examination services performed by consultants. It also does not include diagnostic radiology services and radiation therapy requested by radiologists and radiation oncologists.

Unlike the federal antikickback law, the Stark law does not require intent for a violation. An inadvertent error can thus give rise to liability. The sanctions include refund of amounts billed and collected for the services; civil penalties of up to $15,000 for each bill or claim that the physician knows or should know is a violation; a penalty of up to $100,000 for each referral arrangement or scheme that the physician knows or should know has a principal purpose of effecting forbidden transactions; and a 5-year exclusion from the reimbursement program if the physician knows or should know that a claim is improper.

There are a number of broad exceptions that prevent the statute from effectively prohibiting all financial relationships within the medical community. Each of these exceptions is limited by specific statutory language. Moreover, proposed regulations, if adopted, would narrow the scope of several of these exceptions.[114] The most relevant exceptions are

Physician services. These must be provided or supervised by physicians in the same group practice. "Group practice" is very technically defined and includes (among other things) requirements that substantially all physician-member services be provided through and billed by the group, compensation cannot be based on volume of referrals, and physician-members must provide substantially the full range of that physician's routine services through the group.

In-office ancillary services. The exception applies only within group practices and for services supplied in the same building as the referrer or in another building used for the group's services. This exception does not apply to most kinds of durable medical equipment. Services must be billed by the physician performing the service, by the group practice of that physician, or by an entity entirely owned by that group.

Prepaid plans. Services furnished by HMOs and prepaid plans that have contracted with the government are excluded from the ownership and compensation prohibitions.

113. The 1993 amendments to the Ethics in Patient Referrals Act (the Stark Bill) extended coverage of the law to Medicaid-financed services, thus denying states Medicaid reimbursement for expenditures based on violations of the Stark Act.
114. *See* 57 Fed. Reg. 8588 (1992) (to be codified at 42 C.F.R. pt. 411) (proposed March 11, 1992).

Publicly traded securities. The ownership prohibition does not apply to publicly traded shares of very large corporations.

Certain hospitals. The ownership prohibition does not apply to hospitals in Puerto Rico, entities providing services in designated rural areas, and hospitals if the interest is in the whole hospital and not just a subdivision.

Nonmedical payments. Payments to physicians by hospitals for nonmedical services are not considered a compensation arrangement.

Office and equipment rentals. These are not considered compensation arrangements if the lease is in writing and is for 1 year or more, the property leased is only what is reasonable and necessary for legitimate business purposes and is used exclusively by the lessee (a further exception is made for common office areas), and the charge reflects fair market value and does not take into account the volume or value of referrals.

Employment. This is not a compensation arrangement if it is bona fide. Pay must be for defined services and consistent with fair market value under commercially reasonable terms not related to volume or value of referrals.

Service arrangements. It is not a prohibited compensation arrangement for a physician to contract to provide personal services to an entity under a written agreement that covers all the services, that fulfills and does not exceed legitimate business purposes, that is for 1 year or more, that specifies pay in advance not exceeding fair market value without regard to volume or value of referrals, *and* that does not otherwise violate any law.

Incentive plans. Physicians may be provided with incentives that take referrals into account (e.g., through withholds, capitation, or bonuses) if there is no payment that induces reduction or limit of medically necessary services for any specific patient. The plan must comply with any government regulations if it places the physician or group in "substantial financial risk".[115] Moreover, on demand, the entity must give the government access to determine compliance.

Physician relocation incentives. Compensation arrangements do not include benefits given by hospitals to induce physicians to relocate to the hospital's area in order to join the staff, as long as there is no requirement for referral and any remuneration does not take referrals into account.

---

115. There are no final regulations in place. Under proposed regulations, 57 Fed. Reg. 59024 (1992) (proposed Dec. 14, 1992), substantial risk is a risk of more than 25% of physical compensation. This percentage drops to 15% if the risk assessment or distribution is made more frequently than once a year. The proposed regulations require adequate stop loss on annual patient surveys to ensure adequate satisfaction on access.

Isolated transactions. One-time transactions such as sales of practices are not compensation arrangements if the amount paid is consistent with fair market value without regard to referral volume or value, and if the deal would be commercially reasonable without any referrals.

Hospital group practice arrangements. These are not compensation arrangements if group services are billed by the hospital; the arrangement covers specified inpatient services in writing and is made to comply with government prohibitions against unbundling certain services; it has continued uninterrupted since before 12/19/89; substantially all of the hospital's designated services are provided by the group; and the compensation is consistent with fair market value fixed for units of service in advance without regard to volume or value of referrals in a deal that would be commercially reasonably without any referrals.

Physician payments. Payments *by* physicians are not compensation arrangements if made to laboratories for clinical laboratory services or made to an entity for services consistent with fair market value.

To ease the government's oversight task, the Stark law also requires disclosure to the government of ownership and compensation arrangements. This information will apparently be collected through survey forms and fed into a database maintained by the federal government. Failure to report can result in fines of up to $10,000 per day and program exclusion. Compliance requirements are now being delayed until the government issues report forms and instructions.

False Claims

A number of statutes cover submission of false claims. These statutes may apply to claims made to any payer (public or private), although some are limited to claims submitted to governmental agencies. The options for prosecution are numerous in most jurisdictions but usually fall into one of several categories.

MAIL AND WIRE FRAUD

Federal statutes prohibit the sending of false statements through the mail or by most public telecommunications media.[116] These statutes have been applied to cases ranging from fraud cases to drug conspiracies. In the medical services area they have been successfully applied to billing for imaginary services.[117] An important feature of these statutes is that they

---

116. 18 U.S.C. §1341, 18 U.S.C. §1343.
117. *U.S. v. Hershenow*, 680 F.2d 847 (1st Cir. 1982)

may be applied to fraudulent claims made to private payors (even patients themselves).

A related federal statute, the so-called RICO Act,[118] can also be applied to false medical claims. Although the RICO Act was conceived to combat organized crime, its reach extends far beyond what is traditionally thought of as racketeering. Essentially, it prohibits repeated "predicate" acts such as mail or wire fraud when these are part of the conduct of an enterprise engaged in interstate commerce. The penalties for this are designed to dismantle the enterprise entirely and include prison up to 20 years (or for life if the violation is based on a racketeering activity for which the maximum penalty includes life imprisonment), fines, and forfeiture of the assets used in the enterprise.[119]

FALSE GOVERNMENT CLAIMS

A number of statutes forbid any type of false claim submitted to a government agency. These include:

18 U.S.C. §287—which prohibits false claims against the federal government. This statute relates to requests for reimbursement based on false laboratory results.[120]

18 U.S.C. §1001—which prohibits false statements to a governmental agency. This refers to matters such as research results that do not directly relate to money paid.

18 U.S.C. §286—which prohibits conspiracies to make false claims against the federal government.

31 U.S.C. §3729—which provides for civil liability for knowing submission of a false claim to any government agency or for conspiracy to defraud the government. The penalty is up to $10,000 for each claim plus treble the amount of actual damage caused by the claim. Under this statute, the government only need prove a recklessly false claim, it does not need to prove that you knew the claim was false. In *U.S. v. Krizek*,[121] the federal prosecutor sought $80 million in penalties based on actual false claims of only $245,000!

31 U.S.C. §3802—which provides for a penalty of up to $5000 per violation for the submission of any false, fictitious, or fraudulent claim, any false statement, or any statement that omits material facts.

---

118. 18 U.S.C. §1962 (1984 & 1995 Supp.).
119. 18 U.S.C. §1963 (1984 & 1995 Supp.).
120. *See, U.S. v. Precision Medical Laboratories, Inc.*, 593 F.2d 434 (2nd Cir. 1988).
121. 859 F. Supp. 5 (D.D.C. 1994).

18 U.S.C. §371—which prohibits agreements to defraud the federal government or to commit other offenses (such as wire or mail fraud) if acts are undertaken in furtherance of the agreement.

18 U.S.C. §982 and 1963—which allow the federal government to seize the proceeds of any crime or any property or assets derived from or substituted for the proceeds.

31 U.S.C. §3730—which allows a private person to bring a civil action for a violation of 31 U.S.C. §3729 for the person and for the U.S. Government, in the name of the government.

FALSE PROGRAM-SPECIFIC CLAIMS

42 U.S.C. 1320a-7b (a)—which creates criminal liability for making knowingly false statements in payment submissions for Medicare or Medicaid payment. An example is the conviction in *U.S. v. Naxon*[122] in which a doctor was convicted of seeking payment for work performed by an assistant whom he had not in fact hired and also falsely inflating laboratory bills. Even if you are not personally involved in the billing, you can be convicted if it appears you knew of it and benefited by it.[123]

42 U.S.C. 1320 a-7a—which creates civil liability for making false claims for Medicare or Medicaid payment when the claimant knew or should have known that the claim was false. Penalties include double the amount of the false claim plus $2000 per false claim.

42 U.S.C. 1320 a-7a—which provides for exclusion from the Medicare and Medicaid system for 5 years for patient-related abuse or neglect or for conviction of any Medicare- or Medicaid-related criminal offense.

STATE ENFORCEMENT EFFORTS

Many states have their own antifraud statutes relating to government programs.[124] In several instances, states have passed legislation that also forbids false claims to private payers.[125] Numerous state laws and causes of action create civil or criminal liability for fraudulent claims and statements made in either the public or private reimbursement context. For example, states have larceny laws, fraud laws, and private causes of action for conversion, fraud, misrepresentation, and unfair and deceptive business practices.[126]

122. 940 F.2d 255 (7th Cir. 1991).
123. *See U.S. v. O'Brien, 14 F.3d 703 (1st Cir. 1994).*
124. *See,* e.g., Mass. Gen. Laws c. 118 §40.
125. *See,* e.g., Mass. Gen. Laws c. 175H.
126. *See,* e.g., *Commonwealth v. Arkus Pharm. of Worcester,* 5 Mass. App. Ct. 764, 861 (1977).

Currently, more than 40 states have established Medicaid fraud control units whose job it is to ferret out and prosecute fraudulent program claims.

General Comments

The antifraud laws have tremendous impact on the financial relationships that physicians encounter in the managed care environment.

First, compensation within group practices is now government regulated indirectly through the antireferral requirements. Although it is still possible to share group profits as well as give bonuses for performance, these must be structured so that they have nothing to do with individual decisions to refer within the group. The trick is to find measures of physician value and productivity that focus on the physician's own clinical activities, not upon the residual value of intragroup referrals.[127]

Second, anytime that a physician negotiates a lease with an MCO or sells his or her practice, the antifraud statutes come into play. What the physician sees as a wonderful deal may, in fact, exceed fair market value and thus to fall into a danger zone.

Third, physician financial interests that go beyond the physician group are subject to vigorous scrutiny under the antifraud laws. Thus, arrangements in which the physician owns an interest in a clinic (e.g., through an MSO) may create the appearance of a kickback or may violate antireferral prohibitions unless the relationship meets safe-harbor criteria.

Fourth, the ability of MCOs to recruit and retain physicians may be drastically curtailed by the antifraud laws. The Stark exceptions are largely oriented toward hospitals. Thus, MCOs that are not federally qualified and who want to offer recruiting inducements will have to try to conform to the Stark exceptions for employees, for personal service agreements, and/or for incentive plans. The physician incentive plan exception to Stark permits capitation and other kinds of incentives, but the participants run a risk that the arrangements, in retrospect, will not be seen to be for fair market value.

Fifth, the structure of an MCO itself may create fraud problems. For example, PHOs sometimes have not required more than nominal physician capital investment. Moreover, since physicians may be paid by health care payors directly (on a basis established by the PHO) it may appear that physicians are actually being rewarded for hospital referrals on a per-re-

---

127. Many group practices without walls are struggling to make sure they stay within the law. Because their internal structures are relatively loose, they involve substantial legal risk and must be evaluated very carefully.

ferral basis. In *United States v. Lipkis,*[128] an arrangement by which a clinical laboratory paid a significant service fee to an MSO in exchange for nominal sample collection duties was ruled not to reflect fair market value and thus constituted fraud. The court noted that the agreement was clearly designed as payment for referrals of the MSO's physician business.

Similarly, an MSO that serves physicians by leasing and subleasing space and equipment could create at least the appearance of fraud by negotiating ground leases with a hospital that are too favorable or that involve rebates or payments by the hospital. If the MSO is physician-owned, purchases of practices from physician members are subject to claims that the terms are overgenerous. In fact, MSO ownership of ancillary service providers may create unsolvable problems under the antireferral laws.

GOVERNMENT REGULATION: ANTITRUST

A principal feature of the American economic system is the belief that free competition is a virtue. Starting at the end of the 19th century, Congress began adopting legislation to protect and promote competition among American businesses. Spurred by the activities of the great industrial robber barons, the first federal legislation—the Sherman Antitrust Act of 1890—was enacted to prohibit business practices that distort prices, control markets, or otherwise victimize consumers by suppressing competitive forces.

Antitrust law considerations now permeate virtually the whole American business world. In health care, the market is going through an accelerated frenzy of cost cutting and consolidation. Market forces that until recently only brushed physicians are suddenly being felt acutely. In the push toward managed care, novel business relationships are being developed, and physicians are coming under intense fire for acting in ways that drive health care costs up for consumers. The resulting situation is a minefield of antitrust problems, with the average physician encountering invitations, enticements, and sometimes pressure to enter into relationships that may violate antitrust laws. A basic understanding of these laws and common problems encountered in managed care is therefore important, although any specific situation should be reviewed by an antitrust specialist.

Summary of Selected Federal Antitrust Laws

Most antitrust law is based in federal laws prohibiting monopolies, combinations in restraint of trade, and tying. Many states have laws that

---

128. 770 F.2d 1447 (9th Cir. 1985).

echo the federal laws, although some modify the standards set forth in the federal statutes.[129]

For nonlawyers, the perception of antitrust law is that it is aimed exclusively at monopolies. Section 2 of the Sherman Act (15 U.S.C. §2) does prohibit monopolization or attempts to monopolize. Monopolization is the possession of monopoly power, i.e., the power to exclude competitors, control price, or control output in a "market." Courts will look to a number of factors to determine this power. First and foremost will be market share. If that share is significantly above 50%, a monopoly will very possibly be found. Courts, however, also consider how easy it is for competitors to enter the market and the number and strength of competitors, among other factors, in determining whether a violation exists. Courts also consider whether a competitor is acting willfully to acquire and maintain market power or whether dominance of the market is a result of business skill, legitimate superior business performance, superior products, or luck. Courts consider factors such as control of important technology or production facilities that are used to strangle competition, and predatory pricing schemes.[130]

A key concept in this analysis is the definition of "market." This includes a determination of a relevant product and a relevant geographic area. A hospital may be the only location available for a specific procedure in an area but may not have a monopoly in the relevant market if patients can easily travel out of the area or opt for other procedures that will accomplish the same result.

Despite the public's perception, antitrust violations generally do not involve monopolies. Rather, other sections of the Sherman Act and other federal statues impose antitrust liability for various other types of behavior. For example, Section 1 of the Sherman Act (15 U.S.C. §1) prohibits contracts, combinations, and conspiracies between two or more separate individuals or entities that restrain trade. Because of the requirement that the entities be "separate," a corporation cannot conspire with itself nor can an employee by his or her employment alone be seen as acting in concert with the employer. Furthermore, the courts have recognized that some coordination between a parent and a wholly owned subsidiary is not a "concerted" action.[131]

---

129. A state-by-state review of these statutes is beyond the scope of this chapter. For a compendium review of state antitrust prohibitions; *see* W. J. Haynes, Jr., State Antitrust Laws (1989) and T. M. Wilson, III, *et al.*, Antitrust Federalism: The Role of State Law (1988).

130. This is the practice of setting prices below costs (usually marginal cost) and dumping products or services to destroy competitors and permit later inflated monopolistic pricing to make up for the early losses.

131. *See*, e.g., *Copperweld Corp. v. Independence Tube Corp.*, 467 U.S. 752 (1984).

Section 3 of the Clayton Act (15 U.S.C. §14) prohibits tying and exclusive dealing arrangements involving commodities if the effect may be to substantially lessen competition. In a tying arrangement, the sale of a product or service (the tied product) is conditioned on purchase of another distinct product (the tying product). The concept of "distinct" is crucial. Computers are distinct in many cases from the software they use, but a car body is not distinct from its engine. The existence of a distinction depends not on the relationship between the products but whether there is sufficient demand for the tied product to be sold efficiently apart from the tying product.[132] If the party doing the tying has sufficient economic power in the tying-product market to appreciably restrain competition in the tied market and a not insubstantial amount of commerce in the tied product is affected, the arrangement is presumed to be illegal.

Section 7 of the Clayton Act (15 U.S.C. §18) prohibits mergers, joint ventures, and other acquisition in which the effect may be to substantially decrease competition or to create a monopoly.

Finally, the Federal Trade Commission Act (15 U.S.C. §45) prohibits "unfair methods" of competition and "unfair or deceptive" acts or practices in business. This statute, by far the most potentially far-reaching of all, overlaps each of the other acts.

Jurisdiction for the enforcement of civil or criminal penalties under the Sherman and Clayton Acts rests with the United States Department of Justice. In addition, private parties may bring civil suits under these acts and can in some cases be awarded multiple damages and attorneys' fees. The FTC can enforce the Federal Trade Commission Act through administrative proceedings.

Some Principles of Application

At their most basic level, all contracts decrease competition by requiring parties to engage in business with each other, rather than with competitors. Yet, the antitrust laws are obviously not intended to prevent all contractual relationships. The courts have developed a two-stage analysis for potential violations, allowing transactions to be weighed for their net anticompetitive effect and declaring them illegal only if overall competition is harmed.

THE PER SE RULE

Certain kinds of activity are judged so inimical to competition and so without legitimate business value that they are presumed to be antitrust

---

132. *See Jefferson Parish Hosp. District No. 2 v. Hyde,* 466 U.S. 2, at 19, 21–22 (1984).

violations without further analysis. An example is any agreement to fix prices among competitors. In *Arizona v. Maricopa County Medical Soc'y*,[133] a schedule of maximum suggested fees promulgated by a medical society was deemed *per se* illegal. Another example is a "boycott," which is defined as a concerted refusal by competitors to deal with a business entity. In *In Re Rochester Anesthesiologists*,[134] the defendant anesthesiologists admitted to a *per se* violation of conspiring to reject proposed Blue Cross reimbursement levels in the hope of forcing higher fees. Very few types of activity now are seen to merit this *per se* treatment.

THE RULE OF REASON

Most situations are instead analyzed under a "rule of reason" in which the anticompetitive effects of the action are weighed against the procompetitive benefits. Since even legitimate practices hurt specific competitors, the inquiry is carefully limited to the effects on competition as a whole.

Application of the *per se* and rule of reason standards to entities and arrangements encountered in managed care is still in its infancy. As the marketplace is evolving at breakneck speed, so too will the application of antitrust principles develop rapidly. There currently are, however, several criteria commonly used to evaluate competitive effect in the health care marketplace.

First, federal regulatory agencies will look at the purpose of the venture or arrangement. If the purpose appears to be price fixing or other anticompetitive behavior, violation of the law is almost a foregone conclusion.[135]

In *United States v. Alston*[136] about 50 dentists who were subject to capitation fees with copayments and who had been unsuccessful in individually convincing the insurers to increase fees met, and later many sent letters to the plans requesting higher fees. Three "ringleaders" were indicted. In discussing the strength of the case against them, the court noted that the dentists might have believed they were only complying with insurer requests that they comment on proposed increases in fee schedules and that this would not give rise to criminal liability. Although the court clearly stated that per se illegality would apply to actual agreements to ask for higher fees, it noted

---

133. 457 U.S. 332 (1982).
134. 110 F.T.C. 175 (1988).
135. *See United States v. Massachusetts Allergy Soc'y, Inc.*, 1992–1 Trade Cas. (CCH) §0669, 846 (D. Mass. 1992).
136. 974 F.2d 1206 (9th Cir. 1992)

[m]any things that might occur at a meeting such as in Dr. Alston's office would escape the per se rule and might be perfectly legal under the rule of reason: dentists commiserating over the low fee schedules; or impugning the motivations or integrity of the Plans; even sabre-rattling about economic retribution at some indefinite time in the future if their grievances remain unaddressed. Some such activity, like clamoring for governmental protection of their economic interests . . . would even be constitutionally protected.[137]

Second, in addition to motive, courts and government regulators look at the market power of the actors and of the arrangement. This involves inquiry into the number of competitors in the market, the percentage of competitors who are involved in the venture or arrangement, the venture's exclusivity, and the ability of competing ventures to enter the market.

Third, courts and government regulators will look at the degree to which physician-controlled ventures exclude other physicians. Under current United States Supreme Court precedent, the burden of proving a group boycott against excluded physicians is substantial and must include showing market power or total exclusion from the means of doing business.[138]

Ventures among Physicians

Managed care organizations frequently involve agreements to restrict prices or to otherwise limit competition. When these features are necessary to the venture, they are viewed as ancillary restraints and analyzed under the rule of reason. For example, in *Hassan v. Indep. Practice Associates, P.C.*,[139] the reimbursement system imposed by an IPA on its members was not seen as illegal price fixing since the IPA fulfilled a useful competitive role, a system for reimbursement was necessary for the IPA to exist, and the restraint was outweighed by the competitive utility of the IPA. On the other hand, "sham" provider organizations, in which the financial arrangements and practices of the individual physicians are not truly integrated, can be seen as illegal attempts to allow competing physicians to join together to fix reimbursements.[140]

To help market participants predict the legality of their arrangements, the Department of Justice and the FTC issued a joint statement of en-

---

137. Id. at 1214.
138. *Northwest Wholesale Stationers, Inc. v. Pac. Stationery Printing Co.*, 472 U.S. 284 (1985).
139. 698 F. Supp. 679 (E.D. Mich. 1988).
140. *See Southbank IPA, Inc.*, C-3355, 57 Fed. Reg. 2913 (January 4, 1992).

forcement policy in 1994 (the "1994 Statement").[141] This 1994 Statement has no binding effect on private antitrust lawsuits and does not purport to be the last word on the subject. However, it does provide defined "safety zones" which the regulators believe are acceptable and legal. As with antifraud safe harbors, arrangements not within the safety zones can still be deemed legal, although that legality is not assured. Moreover, qualification in a safety zone does not stop private parties or state prosecutors from bringing antitrust challenges to the practice. Nevertheless, the 1994 Statement provides a reasoned general roadmap to many of the managed care arrangements that a physician will encounter.

The 1994 Statement identifies IPAs, PPOs, and other "physician network joint ventures" as physician-controlled ventures in which the participants agree on prices and other terms of competition and jointly market their services. These arrangements are recognized to provide significant procompetitive benefits for consumers. From the physician's viewpoint, they can result in "decreased overhead, better coverage and more flexible schedules" and can "facilitate referrals and provide visibility."[142]

The 1994 Statement distinguishes between exclusive and nonexclusive ventures. Exclusive ventures restrict the ability of participating physicians to affiliate with others or to work outside the venture. These pose the greatest risk to competition in the market. However, under the 1994 Statement such ventures that contain 20% or less of the physicians who have active admitting privileges in each specialty in the relevant geographic market and that involve substantial risk sharing among physicians are within a safety zone. "Substantial risk" is defined as including a capitated rate plan structure or significant financial incentives internal to the venture to reach specified cost-containment goals. An example is withholding of compensation from all members, with distribution only if goals are met.[143] Capitation and withholds, although mentioned explicitly, are not the exclusive means of achieving such risk sharing.

When the venture is nonexclusive, the safety-zone standard is relaxed to a 30% share of physicians in each specialty with admitting privileges. The 1994 Statement is careful to state that so-called nonexclusive ventures must demonstrate that they are nonexclusive in reality, not just in name. The indicia applied by the federal agencies to test this include

---

141. Statement of Enforcement Policy and Analytical Principles Relating to Health Care and Antitrust, September 27, 1994. See also K. E. Grady, A Framework for Antitrust Analysis of Health Care Joint Ventures, 61 Antitrust L.J. 5765 (1993).

142. N. P. Metenko, Antitrust and Physician Networks 233 (in Health Care Reform and Antitrust at 233 (Practicing Law Institute 1994 New York).

143. The Justice Department has indicated that a 20% withhold is enough to be "substantial." *See* letter 95–6, Mid-South Physician Alliance, Inc., 6 Trade Reg. Rep. (CCH) ¶44,095 at page 43,366 (Mar. 30, 1995). Fifteen percent withholds have received mixed treatment.

The existence of viable competing ventures

Actual physician participation or evidence of physician willingness to participate outside the venture

Substantial revenue earned by venture physicians outside the venture

Absence of evidence of "departicipation" in other ventures

Absence of evidence of coordination by venture physicians in their dealings with other ventures

Even if this "safety zone" is not achieved, the federal regulators will still analyze a venture only under a rule of reason analysis if there is a sharing of substantial risk or the venture allows a new product to be offered. In *Hassan v. Independent Practice Associates*,[144] the court refused to consider whether a physician-owned IPA was engaged in price fixing. The IPA was contracted on a capitated basis to an HMO that withheld 12% of the physicians' fees until a payout at year-end, based on IPA performance. Since IPA members shared the risk of loss and opportunity for profit and since without an IPA, comprehensive physician service for a prepaid fee would not have been available, the court viewed the IPA as a valid and competitively valuable joint venture.

In analyzing the percentage share of market physicians, the government will usually define the market on the basis of specialty. It will include all physicians who are "good substitutes" from the consumer's viewpoint, which involves elements of distance as well as speciality training. The government will then evaluate the potential for suppression of competition in that market, paying special attention to whether the venture can raise prices above competitive levels or prevent entry of competing ventures into the market. If many similar ventures or potentially competing physicians exist in the market, the venture is likely to pass government muster. If there are anticompetitive effects, the government will balance them against procompetitive effects such as increased efficiencies and cost savings (resulting from risk sharing and economics of scale) as well as efficiencies from pooled administrative functions. Finally, the government will consider and balance the effect of any collateral agreements that are "spinoffs" of the venture.

Ventures between Physicians and Other Entities

When dealing with mixed ventures between physicians and other entities (e.g., PHOs), the antitrust analysis changes slightly. Since the most dangerous types of agreements to competition are horizontal (i.e., between com-

---

144. 698 F. Supp. 679 (E.D. Mich. 1988).

petitors in the same stratum of the market),[145] mixed ventures involving vertical relationships among the participants are less likely to raise antitrust concerns.[146] At the same time, some of these vertically mixed ventures are more loosely integrated than physician-only ventures, thus inviting increased antitrust scrutiny.

As set forth in the 1994 Statement, the concept of sufficient integration is important in this context. If integration is insufficient, the *per se* rule may be applied and antitrust illegality could easily be found. If there is little integration, systems have to be built into the venture that will ensure that horizontal elements of the venture will not be seen to collude on price or market allocation.

In the 1994 Statement, the risk-sharing criteria for integration are the same as those for physician-only ventures.[147] If this risk sharing is weak or nonexistent, the venture can still pass government muster by adopting a "messenger model." In this arrangement, competitors in a loosely integrated venture do not communicate with each other about price or terms but with a third-party messenger who then conveys the aggregate information back and forth to other "vertical" elements of the market, such as hospitals or payors. Physicians make individual decisions whether to accept the terms ultimately arrived at.

If the messenger shares data among the physicians, antitrust violations again become a significant concern. The purpose of a messenger system is to prevent horizontal collusion among physicians who have not been sufficiently integrated to avoid antitrust scrutiny.

Because the venture will have a vertical as well as horizontal relationship, the 1994 Statement will also consider the antitrust implications of the vertical elements. If, for example, the vertical contracts in the venture are exclusive, physicians will be prevented from becoming part of competing entities. In *U.S. Healthcare, Inc. v. Healthsource, Inc.,*[148] the court upheld an exclusive dealing clause in an HMO contract because the contract was terminable on 30-days notice and the participating doctors were not significantly restricted. New doctors were constantly entering the market, and the HMO had contracts with only 25% of the state's doctors. The government regulators will look at the effect this type of arrangements has on the ability of competing entities to gain and keep a position in the market. This analysis resembles that applied to exclusive IPAs and PPOs.

---

145. Examples of horizontal arrangements are those among physicians, among hospitals, or among patients.
146. Examples of vertical arrangements are contracts between physicians and hospitals, between hospitals and insurers, and between physicians and patients.
147. If the venture is integrated, the 1994 Statement deems that division of revenue within the venture will not create antitrust problems.
148. 986 F.2d 589 (1st Cir. 1993).

In addition, the 1994 Statement indicates that the government will consider whether the venture excludes physicians (or other providers) under circumstances in which those excluded cannot effectively compete. The government will also recognize procompetitive effects of such exclusions, since they may be useful to ensure competence or ability to meet venture cost-containment goals.

Joint Purchasing Arrangements

To meet managed care goals, care providers (including physicians and hospitals) sometimes enter joint purchasing arrangements. Since these are combinations of buyers, they carry significant antitrust risk. The 1994 Statement recognizes the competitive advantages these arrangements may have, but also the danger of boycotts and price fixing if the joint arrangement can exercise market power or if it can be used to fix so much of the buyers' costs as to allow fixing of resale prices for consumers.

Under the 1994 Statement, joint purchasing arrangements qualify in a safety zone if they account for less than 35% of the total sales of the product or service purchased in the relevant market *and* involve purchase of products or services valued at less than 20% of the total revenue of all products and services sold by each of the competing participants in the arrangement.

In addition, there are several safeguards that may protect arrangements that cannot meet these percentages. The 1994 Statement cites the nonexclusive nature of participation (so that participants can make outside purchases), the use of third-party negotiators, and the confidentiality of each participant's communications to the joint purchasing agent as factors mitigating toward legality.

Factors that mitigate against legality include the inability of excluded competitors to compete effectively without access, and the lack of any significant efficiencies achieved for the participants by the arrangements.

Physician Exchanges of Information

In bargaining with an MCO over a managed care contract, it is desirable for both the MCO and the physician to know what pricing information exists for other physicians as well as for both to have access to medical data and practice standards employed in the physician community. Such information is useful in understanding how to structure and price a physician's managed care relationships.

The 1994 Statement divides this information into fee- and non-fee-related data and further divides it into data that are shared with payors only and information that is shared among providers.

Non-fee-related data, which might consist of practice guidelines or parameters, provides useful information to the public and can sharpen competition by helping the public distinguish between competitors. Sharing this type of information is unlikely to be seen as an antitrust violation unless attempts are made to coerce acceptance of guidelines as standards. If these attempts are made by more than one physician or entity acting in concert, they may be seen as collusion in restraint of trade. An example presented by the 1994 Statement is an agreement by physicians not to provide x-rays to an insurer who wants them before approving payment.

Collective provision by physicians of fee information to MCOs merits stricter scrutiny. Physicians may find themselves as a group providing information on discounts, payment methods, and raw fees to MCOs who are seeking recruits. Among themselves, physicians sometimes find it valuable to share surveys of fees, wages, and benefits so that they can be informed in striking deals with MCOs. If the physicians are already part of an integrated venture, there may be no problem. But, if the physicians are otherwise independent, the danger exists that the "disclosure" will be used as a vehicle to reach consensus on fee levels, i.e., to fix prices. The 1994 Statement defines a safety zone if the information is gathered and communicated by a third party, any fee data shared among physicians are more than 3 months old, individual provider data shared among physicians are hidden as an anonymous statistic with at least five physicians' data supporting each statistic, and no physician's data represent more than 25% of any statistic.

The 1994 Statement warns against collective negotiation by unintegrated provider groups or group threats to boycott purchasers. Explicitly exempted from the safety zone is collective reporting or surveys by physicians of views on future fees and fee-related matters.[149]

---

149. This sharing of prospective fee information will be considered on a case-by-case basis.

□

SECTION FIVE

PERSPECTIVES OF MANAGED CARE

CHAPTER THIRTEEN

THE PROVIDER'S PROSPECTIVE

Thompson H. Boyd III

From the perspective of the provider, nothing has changed the practice of medicine since the arrival of managed care. The change has been enormous in scope. Practicing in the marketplace may be easier when one has a number of issues in focus. These issues fall into four broad categories:

The health care environment
Generalism
Systems improvement
Informatics

THE HEALTH CARE ENVIRONMENT

The number of patients enrolling in managed care plans continues to grow at record levels (1). Patients who have participated in fee-for-service plans are moving in large numbers to the managed care environment, largely through HMOs (health maintenance organizations) and PPOs (preferred provider organizations). Depending on the managed care penetration in a given area of the United States, this movement is seen at various levels of intensity. In 1993, employer-sponsored plans accounted for less than 50% of those insured with traditional indemnity coverage (2).

Because of their interest in controlling costs, managed care plans limit the use of specialists, which can be considered as a "cost center" (3). Copies of referrals generated from the primary care physician are turned in regularly to the managed care company. Data showing the extent of referral use by providers are maintained.

The community as a whole must not be forgotten. Improving public health through governmental programs working in concert with local organizations is needed (4). Incentives for providers to become advocates for the maintenance of health of the public are required (5).

Ethical issues in managed care have been regularly discussed in the medical literature (6). The physician-patient relationship is a delicate balance. Foremost, physicians must look out for the needs of their patients. This trust is essential to the bonding between physicians and patients. However, the physician may receive less financial remuneration with increased utilization of services (laboratory testing, x-ray, referral to specialists). The physician as gate keeper engenders a conflict between serving the patient and conserving resources (7). Guidelines for the allocation of health care in the managed care environment should be established jointly, and there should be an adequate appellate mechanism for disputes and concerns (6). We must maintain a leadership role—advocating the best for our patients and opposing what is not in their best interest (8).

A large population of patients are still uninsured or underinsured (9), yet every citizen should have access to health care. A basic benefit package needs to be provided along with a monitoring system for variations (9).

In some areas of the country, more than 90% of the insured are enrolled in a managed care plan (10). To preserve primary care, it has been advocated that a separate fee schedule be adopted with a revenue floor. Statewide primary care associations must serve as patient advocates during this enrollment phase.

In the office, with students, and on teaching rounds in the hospital, one contemplates what health care will be like by the year 2000. According to Weiner (12), there will be an excess of nearly 165,000 physicians. The supply of primary care physicians will be in balance with the demand, the excess being virtually all specialists. In Connecticut, internist supply is growing faster than the population (22). By the year 2000, 40–60% of Americans will be enrolled in a managed care network (12).

The Council on Graduate Medical Education (COGME) and the American Association of Medical Colleges (AAMC) acknowledge the need to produce more primary care physicians. There is a pressing need for primary care physicians in rural areas and in inner cities. Various models have been proposed. The 50% solution is endorsed by the COGME and AAMC, whereby 50% of all graduating medical students would go into a field of primary care. Others have suggested a 33–67% rule, whereby 33% would go into primary care (13). Clearly a 20–80% model (20% into primary care) would not provide the necessary number of primary care physicians.

COGME and the Physician Review Commission have recommended

that the number of entry-level residency positions be 105% of the number of U.S. medical school graduates (14). The American College of Physicians advocates establishing a National Work Force Commission, which would coordinate fiscal policy for physicians and set manpower goals by determining the adequate number of residency training spots. State and local authorities would provide expertise regarding local needs (15).

Administrative costs in a health system need to be continually reviewed. Abroad, health care expenditures are a fraction of those in the U.S., even under managed care (16).

The job of the primary care provider in preserving the health of patients is multifold. Time is devoted to the acute and chronic medical problems of our patients. Prevention of disease and preservation of wellness are contemporary aspects of the care now provided. Social issues such as poverty, unhappiness, domestic violence, gun control, and substance abuse, which used to be societal issues, are now laid in front of the physician for answers (17). Health involves the ability to handle and deal with these issues in a professional manner.

The quality of medical care can be broken down into technical aspects and interpersonal aspects (18). Clinical outcomes are reflected in the technical aspects, and patient satisfaction in the interpersonal relationship. Physician satisfaction and cost are also involved (19). As a practice grows, with more staff, tasks are broken up into small pieces. Patient satisfaction—generally lower when the organization is larger—reflects access, waiting times, and time with the physician. The more time physicians spend with the patient and answering questions, the more satisfied they are. However, costs tend to decrease as more physicians are added to the practice. They then level off and later increase as the practice grows (U-shaped curve). The ideal size for a practice, in terms of cost and patient satisfaction, needs further study.

In 1965, Congress passed Medicare, legislation that had undergone many years of debate. The uninsured in 1994 constitute a much less powerful group than the elderly in 1965. Health care reform advocates will have to continue to educate the public. It is likely that there will be years of debate before health legislation is agreed upon (20).

Taking care of patients, in the hospital or in the outpatient arena, continues to bring up issues with no easy answers. Physicians employed by managed care organizations have an obligation to their employer. Also, as physicians, they have an obligation to the patient. Case managers, often employed by managed care organizations, interact with primary care physicians and can limit therapeutic options. Potentially, their loyalty can be in conflict—the patient or the employer (21)?

The health team is transcending the boundaries of the hospital. When patients with complex medical problems are discharged, they often need services within hours of their return home. As the length of hospital stays shortens, the patient experiences a cluster of intense services that need to be continued uninterrupted when the patient is at home. The primary care physician remains directly involved with the patients' care and is often in regular contact with the home health agencies. Depending on the locale and medical problem, grant money may be available to support certain home services, such as care for persons with HIV disease. Such patients require intense specialty care in the home. Unfortunately, reimbursement for home care can be finite. As the patient continues to have needs (or as the needs grow), many home agencies are forced to absorb the ongoing costs. Ethically, a number of agencies will not terminate their relationship with the patient because of payment issues.

Physicians need to be more active in the home care field, especially when specialty service are involved. Giving lectures and seminars and participating in other teaching formats will help to unite the team of caregivers. Others will contribute by participating in outpatient therapeutic drug research protocols, such as those involving the protease inhibitors in HIV disease. Research protocols are sponsored by academic institutions, community-based research initiatives, and others.

GENERALISM

The primary care physician is a generalist. Rarely does an issue of a general medical journal appear without an article about generalism. The challenges of everyday life in this field—caring for patients, teaching medical students and residents, working on projects, and keeping up with the literature—are among medicine's biggest. As we train more generalist physicians to care for the patients in our communities, we must pause and consider the richness of the field.

Inhabiting a cluttered world, generalists welcome new information, do not constrict their scope, and have difficulty constructing borders (23). Futility is familiar and not the frustration it can be to specialists. Generalists know a lot about a lot.

The generalist physician provides continuing, comprehensive, and co-ordinated care to a populations of patients with multiple medical problems. The generalist physician must encourage health, promote disease prevention, and use resources efficiently. More generalist scholars are needed to conduct research on the effectiveness of our care and to teach future generalist physicians (30).

With time, primary care physicians get to know many of their patients on deeper levels as they undergo numerous tests and through acute trials of illness. Communication with family members enlightens the patient's narrative. Literary accounts of illness can teach physicians lessons about the lives of sick people and about themselves (24). Narrative skills can help the physician in the setting of quantitative outcomes and yield greater insight into the humor, irony, and conflicts that make up each individual.

Zeldow (25) reported that many medical students knew their specialty choice before the beginning of their third year. A positive experience during the ambulatory rotation can influence a student to choose primary care. Rotations should be done early in medical school (25). At Hahnemann University in Philadelphia, medical students in their first year participate in a number of homeless clinics attended by staff physicians. They also have the opportunity to spend time in a primary care physician's office for several months. This clinical experience enriches the knowledge acquired by reading and studying.

Medical students, residents, and attending physicians should work side by side as a unified team, a vertical linkage between the outpatient office facility and the hospital where acute care is delivered; with decreasing length of hospital stays and higher acuity, the patients' problems and stories will be more likely to be acknowledged as they receive their care (33). This will enhance the formal teaching of the students and residents and portray a realistic approach to the life of a busy internist.

Fourth-year students from Hahnemann University School of Medicine have rotated in our office on monthly rotations for over 4 years. The experience has been complemented by the addition of medical residents who are serving part of their ambulatory rotation. For parts of the year, first-year students are also part of the team. Most patients enjoy having a student (at any level of training) or resident present, and they are examined with the attending. Teaching such a diverse group in the office is invigorating and satisfying.

Other workers (27) found that a student's decision to enter primary care was related to the presence of a Family Medicine Department in the medical school, public status of the school, percentage of public funding, admission preference to students expressing a desire for primary care, and the percentage of in-state students.

Two facts expected to affect the number of general internists include the increasing number of female physicians and international medical school graduates practicing in this country. The women subspecialize at a lower rate, and the foreign national graduates subspecialize at greater rate than U.S. medical graduates (28).

According to the AMA and the AAMC, a graduate medical education–funding pool should be established to support generalist education in which students receive training in the ambulatory care setting and in other programs in the community. Also, incentives need to be developed to encourage more students to go into generalist careers (29).

The primary care physician has an important place in the rural community. The National Health Service Corps was an attempt to bring care to rural and underserved areas. Loan forgiveness and other incentives play a part in recruiting physicians. Innovative student rotations in rural centers will broaden their scope of generalism. Rotations for residents that include experience in patient care, community service, and practice management can provide a balanced view of internal medicine and influence the residents' career choice (71).

The general internist is one who can solve difficult, complex, patient care problems involving multiple organ systems. General internists commonly spend part of the day in the ambulatory care setting and part in the hospital, caring for their patients or acting as medical consultants for another physician's patient. The future general internist will have to reconcile two forces: the wishes of the patient and the limits on health care resources (31). With knowledge and experience in clinical epidemiology, medical ethics, and decision analysis, the patients' interests can be served. A general internist's practice is (a) accessible (easily seen by patients, prompt referral), (b) continuous (patients are followed over time, commonly years, which develops a deep patient-physician relationship), (c) comprehensive (blending of acute and chronic medical problems), and (d) personalized (knowing the patients' belief systems and values, hearing their narrative stories over the years) (24).

Specialists will still be needed to carry on the fundamental research that will be later applied at the bedside. Specialists will also have a role in generalist education (32).

SYSTEMS IMPROVEMENT

A system is a network of interdependent components that work together to accomplish a goal. Without a goal, there is no system (34). In this example, our goal is providing optimal health care to our patients. The system is the current and future health care environment in which we work. All members of the system are involved (42).

Sox has stated that "practice guidelines express one of the noblest aims of medicine: the continuing search for the best way to serve patients" (35). The Institute of Medicine has defined practice guidelines as "systematically developed statements to assist practitioner and patient decisions about appropriate health care for specific clinical circumstances" (36).

In a study in which questionnaires were mailed to American College of

Physicians (ACP) members, familiarity with practice guidelines varied (37). Subspecialists were most accustomed to the guidelines issued by their subspecialty society, and generalists were most familiar with guidelines issued by the ACP. Confidence in ACP guidelines was high, and most agreed that the guidelines were good for advice, education, and improving patient care.

Guidelines must be constructed carefully and revised as new scientific data become available (38). Limiting the scope of a guideline may add to its clarity and usefulness, such as when to add or when to avoid certain interventions (39). Guidelines should be validated by clinical trials; knowing the sensitivity and specificity of a guideline adds to its clinical meaning. Noncompliance with guidelines may not necessarily be related to physician noncompliance, but rather relate to implementation and system inefficiency (40). John Deere and the Mayo Clinic have combined resources and introduced clinical practice guidelines into the electronic information system at the John Deer Family Health Plan in Moline, Illinois, making it easier to follow outcomes (49).

Monitoring how physicians practice medicine is undergoing review. There appears to be little uniformity in how reviews are conducted. An abundance of third-party payers, governmental agencies, and hospitals conduct independent reviews. The ACP (41) has suggested following patterns of care rather than using a case-by-case review. This would include outcomes, costs, and resource consumption.

For the primary care physician, such demands from external entities can be overwhelming. In the last several years, pioneering work in a number of centers in the country has received growing attention. In the presidential address of the Western Thoracic Surgical Association, Fosburg outlines program changes that were enacted at the Scripps Institute (33). "You cannot manage what you cannot measure." Failures are often related to the system design, not the people who try hard and act in good faith (33, 34). Critical pathways were developed consistent with accepted guidelines. The program included family and patient education about the continuum of care from preadmission to postdischarge, evaluation of intervention on outcomes, and charting by exception.

At Scripps, the quality management program is called CareTrac (44). Physicians participating in the program put their patients on a treatment protocol (sometimes called critical path). The clinical CareTrac incorporates accepted guidelines. In 1991–1992, for patients on the CareTrac for DRG 105 (valve replacement without cardiac catheterization), the mean length of stay was 7.4 days (12.3 days for those not on the CareTrac). For DRG 107 (coronary artery bypass graft without cardiac catherization), the mean length of stay was 6.0 days (9.2 days for those not on the CareTrac).

Charges for DRG 106 (coronary artery bypass graft with cardiac catherization were 21% less for those on the CareTrac. Readmission rates, mortality, and morbidity did not worsen under the CareTrac.

The CareTrac is an intervention model, showing that such system changes can lead to improved clinical outcomes (45). Patient satisfaction is elevated as this tool promotes their sense of accomplishment. Costs are reduced, and care is provided more efficiently.

In a managed care setting, patients undergoing surgical treatment for congenital heart disease spent less time in the ICU and had a shorter total length of stay with the use of clinical pathways. No differences were noted in mortality, readmissions, or unscheduled visits (46). Similarly improved outcomes were noted in the elderly undergoing hip replacement. Six-month follow-up of functional status showed that the group on the pathway was actually functioning at a higher level than those not on the pathway (47).

Twenty-four health systems participate in the Consortium Research on Indicators of Systems Performance (CRISP) (48), which collects data about outcomes such as functional status and cost and other indicators such as population health, community benefit, financial performance, and prevention. By sharing data, institutions can compare their performance with that of others.

Clinical pathways are making a difference in patient care (50). Efficient care can be provided and outcomes documented. Responding to the needs of the community in Maryland, health care providers and administrative personnel pulled together and changed the way they provided care, which led to building trust across disciplines. Patients appreciated being told what they were going to experience (51). In another area of the country, health care multidisciplinary personnel in a community hospital reviewed charts, established local guidelines, and outlined a plan of care on a critical path for the treatment of community-acquired pneumonia. They found that when the pathway was followed, the mortality rate decreased from 10.2% to 6.8%, and the average length of stay decreased by 1.3 days, with a 9% reduction in charges (52).

CareMaps or critical pathways reflect the practice patterns of the health care personnel who provide the patient care. The practice patterns should reflect the standard guidelines in the literature, as discussed above. Guidelines may also take into account the best practice or ideal practice in the institution. It is taken for granted that when there are new scientific advances in medicine and technology, the guidelines will change accordingly.

The CareMap or CareMap Tool is a grid that over time describes predicted staff and patient/family behaviors for a defined population, such as asthmatics. "Four essential component of the CareMap Tool are a Timeline, and Index of Problems with Intermediate and Outcome Criteria, a Critical Path, and a Variance Record" (53, 54). Using this tool, care can be provided in a predictable manner, with each knowing what the others will be doing at each stage of the patient's stay in the hospital. Care is monitored and documented systematically. A dynamic and constructive total quality management process evolves. Information can be given back to physicians at regular intervals (such as monthly divisional or department meetings), showing each physician his or her statistics (LOS, cost, patient satisfaction data, specific functional outcome data, etc.). In a confidential manner, physicians can evaluate their performance with respect to other colleagues. With information, physicians can make positive changes leading to more efficient care and have a voice in changing the system for the better.

If physicians take part in constructing the clinical pathways, (physician-generated pathways), they will be able to nurture the pathway and revise it as needed. They will also be able to believe and respect the data it generates. At Hahnemann University, a clinical pathway for asthma was constructed by a panel of physicians, experts, caregivers, and administrative personnel (60). It expected that shortly, 50% of all patients admitted to the hospital will be on a clinical pathway.

Clinical pathways are intended to become part of the medical record. After a new pathway has been used and revised for 12–24 months, key caregivers should be comfortable with it. The pathway should then be part of the medical record. Charting by exception involves actually charting on the pathway and initialing the appropriate area as the care is provided. Deviation from the path must be noted in the patient record. Failure to comply with the pathway is not necessarily bad or negative; but the reason why must be clearly documented and explained in the medical record.

Data generated from the pathways are important and carry strong implications. Managed care organizations are becoming concerned with physicians' outcome data. It will be no surprise for them to desire to interact with physicians who have the better outcome data such as functional outcomes (related to the specific path or DRG), patient satisfaction, cost, and length of stay. Recredentialing and other activities will most likely be affected by the care we provide.

Similarly, hospitals are contracting with managed care organizations. Hospitals need patients, and if the managed care penetration is significant in the local community, the hospital must have contracts. As these come up for review, the hospital will be asked to furnish its outcome data. If this information is not available, talks will cease. With clinical pathways such as the CareMap system, data can be generated efficiently. Computerization of the clinical pathway is now possible in some centers worldwide, making it easier to generate reports.

The state of the art today is the integration of care beyond the four walls of the hospital into the outpatient setting—connecting the entire episode of illness. K. Zander from the Center of Case Management in South Natick, Massachusetts, added the need for a model offering authority and accountability as providers relate to payers (55).

It has been suggested that CareMaps may benefit the defense in a malpractice case by providing the jury with a coherent, coordinate time line of care. When CareMaps are part of the hospital record, they are more likely to be admitted as evidence (46, 57). With the health care team ensuring that guidelines are incorporated into the clinical pathway, one has a powerful tool. When pathways are not used, physicians are still required to incorporate guidelines in their clinical practice. If their practice does not observe recommendations stated in guidelines, they may be held responsible (58). Guidelines can be a two-way street, either supporting the defense or implicating it (59).

INFORMATICS

The generalist physician has to be able to gather and manage information efficiently. In the clinical arena, questions are asked quickly, and answers should be available quickly. The medical literature has become easier to access, and this should be routine when answering consults or discussing patients with other colleagues. Students in the ambulatory setting should be encouraged to answer clinical questions after searching the medical literature in the office.

Since 1986, when Grateful Med was introduced, on-line use has grown from 5,000 to 100,000 accesses per year (61). Access to MEDLINE at the National Library of Medicine can be made via Grateful Med with an account handled by the National Technical Information Service, a part of the U.S. Department of Commerce. Statements are received quarterly. A communications link to one's medical library provides a cost-efficient way to go into MEDLINE, usually at no cost to the user. Another mode of entry to MEDLINE is from PaperChase, found on CompuServe. Physicians' on Line also has access to MEDLINE. The interfaces are becoming more user friendly.

On can use MEDLINE to search for an overview of specific diseases, such as the benefit of cholesterol-lowering medications (62). One can also search about prevention; for example, preventing stoke by use of oral anticoagulants in the setting of nonvalvular atrial fibrillation (63).

Computer diagnostic systems are available; 105 challenging clinical case summaries involving actual patients were prepared by 10 expert clinicians (64). When the data were entered into four computer-based diagnostic systems, the proportion of correct diagnoses ranged from 0.52 to 0.71. Relevant information generated two additional diagnoses per case. There was, however, irrelevant information, and this should be disregarded. This generation of software appears to be a very early attempt at clinical decision making (65), certainly an important step, but there is a lot of room for improvement.

In another study, on a retrospective review of the literature, computer-based clinical-decision support systems had some positive effects on patient outcomes. Improvement was noted in medicine dosing, preventive-care reminder systems, and in areas of quality assurance (74).

Using the computer to access the information found on the Internet is of growing interest. The Internet began in 1969 with the United States Department of Defense–funded ARPANET. In 1986, the National Science Foundation created the NSFNET as a means of linking computers in academic institutions for use in education and research. In 1991, the High-Performance Computing Act was signed, authorizing the construction of a new high-speed computer network, called the National Research and Education Network, that will connect federal agencies with academic institutions and research organizations (66).

Connecting to the Internet requires TCP/IP software on the user's personal computer. Access to the Internet is then through a commercial provider, a number of which have flourished in the last several years. A basic account involves having a shell account in which you use a terminal program. SLIP or PPP accounts offer the user a greater variety of services; one is directly on the Internet and can use graphically based programs. Other modes of entry include connection to a computer that is already an Internet host or via an on-line service such as CompuServe, Prodigy, America Online, GEnie, or Delphi (69).

The primary care provider can do a number of functions on the Internet. Electronic mail allows one to communicate with colleagues all over the world. An Internet address can be obtained from the commercial provider or the institution where you gain Internet access. Electronic discussion lists are available. Mailing lists about various topics have evolved into USENET groups. This is part of what some term the virtual community.

Early applications of the Internet included Telnet, in which the uses actually takes control of a remote computer. The file transfer protocol (FTP) allows transfer of files across the Internet. Later functions included using gophers—menuing systems allowing the user to select specific files and programs—developed at the University of Minnesota. Linking gopher sites allows one access to an array of information on the Internet. An index of gopher information can be found in a resource called Veronica. Archie is a system for locating specific files. WAIS (wide-area information server) indexes large text files and documents.

The worldwide web (WWW) offers an array of information, including text, sound, and graphics. Files written in the hypertext (HTML) format are accessed, and navigation through the WWW is made possible with programs such as Mosaic and Cello. The WWW was created by the European Laboratory for Particle Physics (CERN) in Geneva, Switzerland. Mosaic was developed at the National Center for Supercomputing Applications at the University of Illinois–Urbana. The need for interfaces that find and link information is being addressed by the Unified Medical Language System Project (75).

Medical applications of the Internet were recently reviewed (66–68). A number of USENET discussion groups and mailing lists are available to users. Many medical center are gopher sites containing information such as the Centers for Disease Control and Prevention's Morbidity and Mortality Weekly Report. Other information is supplied by the NIH and the FDA. Medical centers with gopher servers include the University of Southern California and the University of California at San Francisco (68).

OncoLink from the University of Pennsylvania can be reached by gopher (cancer.med.upenn.edu) or WWW (http://cancer.med.upenn.edu). Other areas that can be reached either by gopher or WWW include the Johns Hopkins University, National Institutes of Health, National Library of Medicine, and World Health Organization (68).

With telecommunications technology, physicians in rural areas experience less isolation. Barriers of time and distance erode when physicians in rural areas can interact with other colleagues and can maintain their skills and medical acumen through continuing medical education activities (70).

Other clinical advances invigorating the rural experience include consultative point-to-point digital/audio interactive sessions with physicians in other institutions. Patients can be viewed by the on-line consultant. X-ray and pathology slides can be a topic of discussion and learning (73). Students at the University of Mexico assigned 2-month rotations with community preceptors were provided with computers with links to MEDLINE (Grateful Med and Lonesome Doc). Access to other databases throughout Internet was provided. The fruit of the experience was that 25% of the students accepted positions in rural areas (72).

Computerization of the medical record has been a slow process (61). LDS Hospital at the University of Utah has integrated the clinical departments in the institution. They have found that nearly every department needs to have information provided by another department—such as age, sex, height, weight—made available to the pharmacy, laboratory, and physicians. With information accessible to others, there will be some loss of privacy.

Natural language processing has the potential to extract clinical data from narrative reports (78). In coding diagnoses from chest radiographs, the language-processing software did as well as radiologists. Notes and textual reports from patient visits contain untapped sources of clinical data. As such work matures and is refined, it will be an important contribution to the electronic medical record (79).

When asked about the grand challenges of the field of medical Informatics, information from the American College of Medical Informatics' listserv contained a number of items, including a complete computer-based patient record, automatic coding of free-text reports, histories, discharge summaries, automated analysis of medical records, a uniform user interface, and a clinical-decision support system (80).

Primary care providers must be familiar with, and active in, the design of the clinical computer systems. These tools are becoming the center point of the practice of medicine. They will allow us to deliver more efficient and better care for our patients. Functional outcomes will be recorded and serve as a barometer of the kind of care we deliver. Functional outcomes, patient satisfaction data, and utilization of resources should be documented by case types with tools such as CareMaps.

Physicians need to be part of their institutional informatics committee. As the hospital computer system expands, physicians' input is needed. The system must be able to tie in with the physicians' offices. Data available in the hospital should be seamlessly available in the physician's office. The physician's office is the front line of medical care. The informatics committee should be multidisciplinary, including information service, administrative, clinical, and legal representatives.

Open discussions regarding the confidentiality of the computerized medical record should occur early in the process (81). The system must track which individuals have requested access to specific information, to ensure security. Users should only be able to access information they need and be restricted from areas in which they have no business. Over 60 individuals can be expected to access a patient's record during the course of an average stay (82). Third-party payers have access to medical records. Policies on overriding access barriers in patient emergencies have to be created.

The computerized medical record has taken on a larger scope for some: the lifetime medical record. This would contain inpatient data, outpatient data, and demographic information over the span of many years or a lifetime. How much data should be included? Will the results of every laboratory test, results of every x-ray be recorded? Who will choose what is to be included and excluded?

The primary care physician will have to deal with these issues when the systems are in place. It is important for the primary care physician to get in on the ground floor and play an active role in policy making and systems design.

REFERENCES

1. Iglehard JK. Health policy report. Physicians and the growth of managed care. New Engl J Med 1994;331:1167–1171.
2. Gabel J, Liston D, Jenson G, Marsteller J. The health insurance picture in 1993: some rare good news. Health Aff (Milwood) 1994;13(1):327–336.
3. Kassirer JP. Access to specialty care [editorial]. New Engl J Med 1994;331:1151–1153.
4. Baker EL, Melton RJ, Stange PV, et al. Health reform and the health of the public. Forging community health partnerships. JAMA 1994;272:1276–1282.
5. Fielding J, Halfon N. Where is the health in health system reform? JAMA 1994;272:1292–1296.
6. Council on Ethical and Judicial Affairs, American Medical Association. Ethical issues in managed care. JAMA 1995;273:330–335.
7. Pellegrino ED. Rationing health care: the ethical of medical gatekeeping. J Contemp Health Law Policy 1986;2:23–45.
8. Clancy CM, Brody, HB. Managed care. Jekyll or Hyde [editorial]? JAMA 1995;273:338–339.
9. Council on Ethical and Judicial Affairs, American Medical Association. Ethical issues in health care system reform, the provision of adequate health care. JAMA 272;1994:1056–1062.
10. Pulley M. Northern California: crucible of change. Integrated Health Care Rep 1993; Dec:1.
11. Alper PR. Primary care in transition. JAMA 1994;272:1523–1527.
12. Weiner JP. Forecasting the effects of health reform on US physician workforce requirement. Evidence from HMO staffing patterns. JAMA 1994;272:222–230.
13. Cooper RA. Seeking a balanced physician workforce for the 21st century JAMA 1994;272:680–687.
14. Council on Graduate Medical Education. Fourth report: recommendations to improve access to health care through physicians workforce reform. Washington, DC: US Department of Health and Human Services, January 1994.
15. Ginsburg JA, Scott HD. A national health work force policy. Ann Intern Med 1994;121:542–546.
16. McDermott J. Evaluating health system reform. The case for a single-payer approach. JAMA 1994;271:782–784.
17. Fitzgerald FT. The tyranny of health. New Engl J Med 1994;331:196–198.
18. Donabedian A. Explorations in quality assessment and monitoring, vol II. The criteria and standards of quality. Ann Arbor, MI: Health Administration Press, 1982.
19. Barr DA. The effects of organizational structure on primary care outcomes under managed care. Ann Intern Med 1995;122:353–359.
20. Blumenthal D. Health care reform—past and future. New Engl J Med 1995;332:465–468.
21. Rodwin MA. Conflicts in managed care. New Engl J Med 1995;332:604–607.
22. Douglass AB, Hinz CF. Projections of physician supply in internal medicine: a single-state analysis as a basis for planning. Am J Med 1995;98:399–405.
23. Lee RV. The jaundiced eye: generalism in general: Am J Med 1995;98:304–305.
24. Charon R, Banks JT, Connelly JE, et al. Literature and medicine: contributions to clinical practice. Ann Intern Med 1995;122:599–606.

25. Zeldow PB, Preston RC, Daugherty SR. The decision to enter a medical specialty: timing and stability. Med Educ 1992;26:327–332.
26. Fincher RME, Lewis LA, Jackson TW. Why students choose a primary care or nonprimary care career. Am J Med 1994;97:410–417.
27. Martini CJM, Veloski JJ, Barzansky B, Xu G, Fields SK. Medical school and student characteristics that influence choosing a generalist career. JAMA 1994;272:661–668.
28. Lyttle CS, Levey GS. The National Study on Internal Medicine: XX. The changing demographics of internal medicine residency training programs. Ann Intern Med 1994;121: 435–441.
29. Cohen JJ, Todd JS. Association of American Medical Colleges and American Medical Association joint statement on physician workforce planning and graduate medical education reform policies. JAMA 1994;272:712.
30. Kimball HR, Young PR. A statement on the generalist physician from the American Boards of Family Practice and Internal Medicine. JAMA 1994;271:315–316.
31. Sox HC, Scott HD, Ginsburg JA. The role of the future general internist defined. Ann Intern Med 1994;221:616–622.
32. Training in subspecialty internal medicine. On the chessboard of healthcare reform. Association of Subspecialty Professors. Ann Intern Med 1994;121:810–813.
33. Harris ED. Morning report [editorial]. Ann Intern Med 1993;119:430–431.
34. Deming WE. The new economics. Cambridge MA: Institute of Technology Center for Advanced Engineering Study, 1993.
35. Sox H. Practice guidelines: 1994 [editorial]. Am J Med 1994;97:205–207.
36. Institute of Medicine Committee to Advise the Public Heath Service on Practice Guidelines. Clinical practice guidelines: directions for a new agency. Washington, DC: National Academy Press, 1990.
37. Tunis SR, Hayward RSA, Wilson M, et al. Internists' attitudes about clinical practice guidelines. Ann Intern Med 1994;120:956–963.
38. Dans PE. Credibility, cookbook medicine, and common sense: guidelines and the college. Ann Intern Med 1994;120:966–968.
39. McDonald CJ, Overhage JM. You can follow and can trust. An ideal and an example [editorial]. JAMA 1994;271:872–873.
40. Ellrodt AG, Conner L, Riedinger M, Weingarten S. Measuring and improving physician compliance with clinical practice guidelines. A controlled intervention trial. Ann Intern Med 1995;122:277–282.
41. Audet AM, Scott HD. The oversight of medical care: a proposal for reform. Position paper. Ann Intern Med 1994;120:423–431.
42. Schiff GD, Bindman AB, Brennan TA. A better quality alternative JAMA 1994;272:803–808.
43. Fosburg RG. Fulfilling expectations. J Thorac Cardiovasc Surg 1993;103:194–200.
44. Trubo R. If this is cookbook medicine, you may like it. Med Econ March 22, 1993.
45. Campbell AB, Lakier NS. Process of intervention—applying TQM to clinical care. Healthcare Forum J 1992;Jul/Aug:82–83.
46. Turley K, Tyndall M, Roger C, et al. Critical pathway methodology: effectiveness in congenital heart surgery. Ann Thorac Surg 1994;58:57–65.
47. Ogilvie-Harris DJ, Botsford DJ, Worden Hawker R. Elderly patients with hip fractures: improved outcome with the use of care maps with high-quality medical and nursing protocols. J Orthop Trauma 1993;7:428–437.
48. Bergman R. Are my outcomes better than yours?. Hosp Health Networks, Aug 5, 1994.
49. Dazé CJ. Mayo Deere to beyond guidelines to wider management of diseases. Managed Care 1994;Aug:4950.
50. Headrick LA, Neuhauser D. Quality health care. JAMA 1995;273:1718–1720.
51. Lumsdon K. Architects of care. Hosp Health Networks, March 20, 1994.
52. McGarvey RN, Harper JJ. Pneumonia mortality reduction and quality improvement in a community hospital. QRB 1993;19:124–130.
53. Zander K. Critical pathways. In: Melum M, Sinioris M, eds. Total quality management. Chicago: American Hospital Association Publishing, 1992;305–314.

54. Zander K, ed. Managing outcomes through collaborative care. The application of care mapping to case management. Chicago: American Hospital Publishing, 1995.
55. Lumsdom, K. Beyond four walls. Hosp Health Networks 1994;5 Mar:44–45.
56. Nolan C. An analysis of the use and effect of CareMap tools in medical malpractice litigation. South Natick, MA: Center for Case Management, 1994.
57. Lumsdon, K. Clinical paths: a good defense in malpractice litigation? Hosp Health Networks, July 5, 1994.
58. Felsenthal E. Doctors' own guidelines hurt them in court. Wall Street Journal, October 19, 1994.
59. Hyams AL, Brandenburg JA, Lipsitz SR, Shapiro DW, Brennan TA. Practice guidelines and malpractice litigation: a two-way street. Ann Intern Med 1995;122:450–455.
60. Bean B, ed. Mapping care. Issues Outcomes 1995;1:3–4.
61. Lindberg DAB, Humphreys BL. Computers in medicine. JAMA 1995;273:1667–1668.
62. Oxman AD, Cook DJ, Guyatt GH. Users' guides to the medical literature. VI. How to use an overview. JAMA 1994;272:1367–1371.
63. Guyatt GH, Sackett DL, Cook DJ. Users' guides to the medical literature. II. How to use an article about therapy or prevention. JAMA 1994;271:59–63.
64. Berner ES, Webster GD, Shugerman AA, et al. Performance of four computer based diagnostic systems. New Engl J Med 1994;330:1792–1796.
65. Kassirer JP. A report card on computer-assisted diagnosis—the grade: C [editorial]. New Engl J Med 1994;330:1824–1825.
66. Glowniak JV, Bushway MK. Computer networks as a medical resource. Accessing and using the Internet. JAMA 1994;271:1934–1939.
67. NcKinney WP, Barnas GP, Golub RM. The medical applications of the Internet: informational resource for research, education, and patient care. J Gen Intern Med 1994;9:627–634.
68. Glowniak JV. Medical resources on the Internet. Ann Intern Med 1995;123:123–131.
69. Ayre R. Making the Internet connection. PC Magazine 1994;13:118–184.
70. Weiner J. Rural primary care. Ann Intern Med 1995;122:380–390.
71. Philbrick JT, Connelly JE, Corbett EC, Ropka ME, Pearl SG, Reid RA, et al. Restoring balance to internal medicine training: the case for the office teaching practice. Am J Med Sci 1990;299:43–49.
72. Scaletti J. Telecommunication and rural health communities [editorial]. Ann Intern Med 1995;122:379.
73. Taylor KS. We're (almost) all connected. Hosp Health Networks 1994:42–47.
74. Johnston ME, Langton KB, Haynes RB, Mathieu A. Effects of computer-based clinical decision support systems on clinical performance and patient outcome. A critical appraisal of research. Ann Intern Med 1994;120;135–142.
75. Lindberg DAB, Humphreys BL, McCary AT. Unified medical language system. Methods Inf Med 1993;32:281–291.
76. Gardner RM. Integrated computerized records provide improved quality of care with little loss of privacy. J Am Med Inform Assoc 1994;1:320–322.
78. Hripcsak G, Friedman C, Alderson PO, DuMouchel W, Johnson SB, Clayton PD. Unlocking clinical data from narrative reports. A study on natural language processing. Ann Intern Med 1995;122:681–688.
79. Tierney WM, Overhage JM, McDonald CH. Toward electronic medical records that improve care. Ann Intern Med 1995;122:725–726.
80. Sittig DF. Grand challenges in medical informatics [editorial]? J Am Med Inform Assoc 1994;1:40–41.
81. Andresen DC. The computerization of health care: can patient privacy survive? J Health Hosp Law 1993;26:1–10,19–20.
82. Waller AA, Fulton DK. The electronic chart: keeping it confidential and secure. J Health Hosp Law 1993;26:104–109.

CHAPTER FOURTEEN

THE MEDICAL
DIRECTOR'S PERSPECTIVE

Harry Gottlieb and J. Thomas Danzi

The traditional role of a medical director has been to represent the medical staff's views to administration and to facilitate the medical staff's compliance with institutional and external agencies' policies and regulations. The function of a medical director has changed with the increased penetration of managed care into the marketplace. The medical director's view can now include contract negotiations, clinical resource utilization review in both the inpatient and ambulatory settings, clinical outcome measurement and management, and clinical information systems. The new responsibilities are appropriate whether the medical director represents a managed care company or a health care provider institution but will be prioritized differently depending on the stage of penetration of managed care in the local market.

An important function of a hospital or medical group practice medical director is to educate the medical staff about the important differences between managed care and traditional indemnity health insurance coverage. Knowing managed care's definition, philosophy, contractual implications, and assessment of a provider's care is important. The medical director must gain the provider's acceptance of the importance of clinical outcome assessment and the development and implementation of clinical guidelines and pathways. The medical staff of either type of health care institution should assume the leadership of the latter processes to ensure their success. The essential role that clinical resource utilization review has in the new paradigm of health care delivery requires its acceptance by physicians.

The medical director's ability to educate the medical staff about the importance of population-based health maintenance compared with the treatment of individuals with disease is also of strategic value to the organization. This may represent the medical director's greatest challenge, since medical school and postgraduate educational training has typically not prepared physicians for this important change and the American public now has its greatest awareness of wellness and health maintenance.

As people become increasingly knowledgeable about health care provision and wellness, their need for greater participation in the decisions relative to their health care increases. Hospitals are addressing this need with new patient-focused care delivery models and enhanced patient education tools. Unfortunately, most physicians have not adjusted their patient-physician relationships to a mutually informed process that satisfies their patients' needs. Medical directors are responsible for educating their medical staffs about the requirements of their new patient relationships as well as the legal and ethical implications of informed consent with a more health care–educated population. The medical director's leadership is important to effectively promote the medical staff's acceptance of the institution's patient focused-care programs.

As physicians enter into contractual relationships with managed care companies, a medical director can be an excellent informational resource on the new glossary of terms in these contracts. What is the significance of a "bundled" or "carve-out" agreement for the institution and providers? What risk pools does the contract have? What features are addressed in the patient satisfaction questionnaire? How does the cap rate per enrollee compare with the institutional and provider's average cost per visit? The answers to these questions will determine to some degree the success of health care teams in a managed care–dominant market.

The perspective for a medical director at an academic medical center is different because of the organizational differences at these institutions. The imminent role of the dean and chairpersons permits the medical director to facilitate both the educational needs of the faculty and the managed care contractual negotiations. The challenges faced by most academic medical centers to become competitive in the managed care market has forced these institutions into novel strategies to strengthen their economic foundations (1, 2). Faculty acceptance of these nontraditional approaches has involved some reservation in most universities. Expansion of the primary care departments and creation of networks to secure managed care contracts has decreased available resource allocation to the subspecialists. The apparent shifts in the power base of the fiefdoms in these academic institutions has caused concern for the traditional-thinking faculty member.

A medical director can be of valuable assistance as these institutions evaluate their present methods of faculty compensation. As more of their income becomes based on capitated or discounted fee agreements, these institutes must teach their faculty the differences between fee-for-service and capitated agreements. The paradigm in health care reimbursement has shifted from "more is better" to "appropriate is right." The associated changes in how the departments are compensated by the payers will force a reevaluation of faculty compensation. They could result in lower base salaries for the specialists and a higher base salary with incentive clause agreement for the primary care faculty. The resulting dichotomy with the present method of compensating faculty will result in interesting meetings between departments, chairs, and deans.

A medical director for a managed care company will have different challenges, depending on the stage of managed care penetration in the marketplace. The medical director's role in an mature market might include provider recruitment to the plan, educating the practitioners about providing care in managed care environment, and ensuring that providers have the data necessary to effect changes in their practice style. As the managed care market matures, the medical director's functions might include developing quality and outcome indicators for the plan, securing an agreement for subspecialist capitation, and resolving of enrollee concerns about the plan's coverage or provider's care.

Most medical directors believe that managed care can improve the health of the American public and provide health care more efficiently. Some fear that the predominant process seems to involve management or steerage of patients rather than management of care. The minority of medical directors are awaiting outcomes data (other than cost information) that confirm the value of this new approach to health care on the public's health. The medical director's perspective should be considered within the context of his or her personal view and that of the employer.

The medical director can address the ethical considerations that managed care present to providers and payers; for example, issues relating to the patient-physician relationship and the allocation of health care resources by the plan (3, 4). The managed care industry must become accountable for the health outcomes of its enrollees, not just a positive bottom line (5). Until it is proven that managed care can give more for less, relative to the long-term health of its enrollees, the corporate profit margin should be lower so that more health care money can be allocated to the patient-provider relationships.

REFERENCES

1. Inglehart JK. Rapid changes for academic medical centers. N Engl J Med 1994;331:1391–1395.

2. Iglehart JK. Rapid changes for academic medical enters. N Engl J Med 1995;332:407–411.
3. Emanuel EJ, Dubler NN. Preserving the physician-patient relationship in the era of managed care. JAMA 1995;273:323–328.
4. American Medical Association. Ethical issues in managed care. JAMA 1995;273:330–335.
5. Clancy CM, Brody H. Managed care. Jekyll or Hyde? JAMA 1995;273:338–339.

CHAPTER FIFTEEN

THE MEDICAL STUDENT'S PERSPECTIVE

Carolyn L. Danzi

Needed change in the health care delivery system of this country has been discussed since the latter half of my high school years. While applying to college, I was aware of the concern about the cost of health care, the application of high technology in the diagnosis and treatment of disease, and the increased use of utilization review techniques by health care payers. At this time, my father was employed as a subspecialist in a large multispecialty group practice. Many discussions with family or friends centered on the changes that were occurring or would occur in the health care delivery system. Frequently, these discussions made me reconsider my career choice of medicine because of how the practice of medicine would be changed.

Throughout my collegiate years, I tried to keep updated on the status of health care reform. During these years, I became aware of the emergence of managed care as a prominent factor in the health care markets of several metropolitan regions in this country, and the impact of the health maintenance movement in California on the careers of family friends became evident. The impact seemed to be greater on specialist practices than on those of primary care physicians. Many "gatekeepers," as they referred to themselves, seemed content with their new practice style and were excited about the preventive health aspects that health maintenance organizations (HMOs) offered to their enrollees. The discussions of the potential changes in lifestyles and incomes that would result from this managed care movement seemed realistic and frequently resulted in the advice that if I was considering a career in medicine, I should research the opportunities that will exist in one of the primary care specialty areas.

My first 2 years of medical school passed very quickly, with little time to worry about the implications of managed care and health care reform to my professional career. After my first year of clinical medicine, I received much advice from the clinical service coordinators to whom I was assigned. This followed three general themes. The first was to choose a primary care career because of the eminent role that these physicians will have in a managed health care delivery system. The second related to the probability of greater financial reward for primary care providers than for subspecialists. The last was to practice or provide high-quality, cost-effective medical care that was appropriately documented.

As I prepare for the second phase of my medical board examination, I feel quite comfortable with my clinical medicine knowledge base. Unfortunately, I feel inadequately prepared in the skills and knowledge to practice in a managed health care delivery system. The present curriculum at most medical schools does not teach the important differences between traditional indemnity health insurance and prepaid or managed care health insurance or the importance of clinical outcomes measurements and clinical pathways application within this new paradigm of health care delivery.

Medical schools need to ensure that their graduates are properly positioned to provide appropriate efficient care in the 21st century. There should be lectures on health care policy, medical information systems, quality or performance improvement, health care team concepts, individual practice and management skills, the ethics of managed care, utilization review, the economics of managed care/fee-for-service medicine, and contract agreements for both types of health care coverage. It is no longer acceptable for medical school graduates to be trained to practice medicine by the standards of the late 1970s and early 1980s in the fee-for-service health care delivery system (1).

It takes years to effectively change the curriculum at a medical school. As I took my rotations during senior year, I could see that the traditional clinical medicine education that occurs in most academic medical center clinics is not compatible with effective health care delivery under a capitated agreement (2, 3). The practice of having a student or resident evaluate the patient, discuss the care with the attending, and finally, evaluate the patient with the attending is not time effective for the number of enrollees who must be evaluated under a managed care contract. The situation will become more difficult as more Medicare and Medicaid HMOs are formed. The faculty must learn to practice effectively within this new paradigm of health care yet acquire new educational skills to educate the students in clinical medicine. Without these essential changes, the academic medical centers will continue "under siege" (4).

The medical schools and academic medical centers prospered under the medical technology expansion of the 1970s and 1980s, with increased numbers of faculty and the acquisition of expensive diagnostic and therapeutic equipment. It will be difficult for these institutions to become cost comparative within a market-driven managed health care delivery system. They may be limited in the future to providing research and selected subspeciality areas of health care (5). We can not allow the competitive marketplace to preclude the research that is necessary for new medical discoveries. The concern is whether such limitations would affect the ability of the academic medical centers to train primary care physicians.

It is likely that I will be practicing pediatrics for a group practice in the future. This group may be independent or owned by a managed care company. Under either scenario, my income will depend upon my ability to provide high-quality, cost-effective health care that benefits both the enrollees and the managed care insurance company. Because my education and training will benefit not only me but also the health care insurance company, I believe that the health insurance companies must share financial responsibility for medical education with the federal government (6, 7).

As a new graduate, I am filled with idealism and excitement about providing health care. I am hopeful that the academic medical centers will be able to make the necessary changes to ensure their continued importance in the health care delivery system of this country. I am idealistic enough to hope that the managed care insurance companies will share the responsibility of the cost of educating their future health care providers. The new leadership of the federal government must ensure that any health care reform legislation addresses these two important topics.

REFERENCES

1. Sabin J. Clinical skills for the 1990's. Hosp Community Psychiatry 1991;42:605–608.
2. Barzansky B, Perloff J. Medical education in prepaid settings. Educ Health Professions 1989;12:300–312.
3. Barzansky B, Perloff J. Trends in the use of outpatient settings for medical education. In: Flexner B, ed. [title?] New York: Greenwood Press, 1992:129–140.
4. Kassirer JP. Academic medical centers under siege. N Engl J Med 1994;331:1370–1371.
5. Inglehart J. Rapid changes for academic medical centers. N Engl J Med 1994;331:1391–1395.
6. Moore GT. Health maintenance organizations and medical education. Academic Med 1990;65:427–432.
7. Moore GT. Perspective and prospectives for HMO's in medical education. HMO Pract 1988;2:122–124.

CHAPTER SIXTEEN

AN APPROACH FOR SUCCESS

Joseph R. Carver

"It was the best of times, it was the worst of times" (1). For the physician approaching the end of the 20th century, a more accurate description of the United States health care system is not possible. New technology, genetically engineered drugs, gene therapy, and advanced noninvasive diagnostic capabilities all contribute positively to the excitement of medical practice. A focus on cost containment, loss of autonomy, a fear of income reduction, and economic credentialing have produced a fear of imposed change and questionable future survival. In the midst of this complex dichotomy how can physicians continue to thrive? What strategic decisions must be made today? What tools must be developed to not only remain viable but also to deliver high quality care at an affordable cost? Future economic restraint will not continue to allocate one of every eight dollars spent in this country to health care. Future health care delivery will be dominated by some form of managed care.

CURRENT ENVIRONMENT AND FUTURE TRENDS

In 1995, health care is responsible for 13% of the gross national product of the United States. In 1994, 20% of the population was insured under some form of managed care; an increase from 14.9% in 1991. This progressive growth has developed largely at the expense of traditional indemnity coverage and now includes the Medicare and Medicaid populations (2, 3).

Although there is regional variation in the activity, maturity, and impact of managed care (4), several trends that dominate each marketplace relate to finances, medical practice, care delivery, and physician accountability. To understand how to prepare for the future, it is necessary to understand their influence in relation to physician behavior, decision making, and posturing for the future. In broad terms, the issues are listed in Table 16.1 and are discussed below.

Table 16.1
Current Environment and Future Trends

Application of classic economic rules to the practice of medicine and health care
Capitation and risk assumption
Formation of networks
Regionalization of "high-tech" "high-cost" services
Shift of service site from inpatient to outpatient
Use of nonphysician caregivers
Shift in paradigm to being proactive, and population management and the
standardization of care through clinical pathways
An implied overabundance of specialists

Application of Classic Economic Rules to the Practice of Medicine and the Delivery of Health Care

Currently, the practice of medicine does not follow the same economic rules as the rest of the business world. Significant differences reviewed by Tiesberg et al. (5) include

1. Consumers (patients and physicians) do not have a financial stake in what they purchase; i.e., the cost is generally the responsibility of a third party. They are not the payers. Given the choice between a Rolls Royce and a Volkswagen Beetle, who would take the latter if somebody else is paying?
2. Consumers do not purchase care on the basis of objective measures of outcomes or quality, they do not usually comparison shop, and they have no idea of the relationship between price and quality for a purchased treatment or procedure. This truth approaches 100% when applied to emergency situations. Because of this, some suppliers (doctors and hospitals) have remained economically successful charging more than a competitor for equal or even lesser quality.
3. Prices have continually risen faster than the general cost of living increase, remaining high even in the presence of excess capacity. The laws of supply and demand have not applied.
4. Physicians and hospitals never had the incentive or need to refer or purchase services (i.e., laboratory studies, x-rays, or specialist consultation) from a more cost-competitive, less expensive, or more cost-efficient vendor;
5. Irrational duplication is unchecked and not governed by market forces.

Managed care is "healing" this economic illness in medical care delivery. These deviations from the "laws" that govern other businesses are slowly being restored to match the rest of the business world. Understanding that the future business of medicine will more closely resemble the real world of business in which success follows classic economic theory is crucial for any practice reorganization or posturing decisions that are made today. Supply and demand rules will apply; purchasers will look to "Medicine Consumers Report" to pick a doctor or ancillary service that will be accountable for cost and quality. The first major step in preparing for the future is acknowledging that the current chaotic application of the laws of economics is ending rapidly.

Capitation and Ultimate Risk Assumption

Many payment models have been suggested to replace the current fee for service system. They include

1. "Fee for time," in which payment is based on a relative time value for each type of encounter. There is recognition of cognitive interventions and a devaluation of testing (6).
2. "Fee for benefit," in which payment is based on the outcome and long-term benefit of a procedure. For example, the reimbursement for coronary artery bypass surgery would be more for a 40-year-old male with unstable angina and left main disease than for an 80-year-old male with lung cancer and single right coronary artery disease (7).
3. Case rates or episodes of care, in which a single all-inclusive payment is made for a defined time period based on a diagnosis, an all-inclusive DRG for all sites of care; for example, $100 for the x-ray evaluation of a headache or $400 for the 4-month treatment and evaluation of chest pain.
4. Capitation, which pays a fixed amount of money on a regular basis for the care of a defined population. The dollar figure is independent of the type or quantity of the services rendered.

Capitation is the most likely survivor of this group and the model for payment in the future. It represents a dramatic change from the fee-for-service world that presently dominates reimbursement. Initial success and long-term viability for physicians are based on understanding and accepting a new mind-set for clinical management. Success in this new world will be proportional to the provider's knowledge and ability to respond to this change. Before making any decisions about entering into a capitated arrangement, the following minimum knowledge base and approaches are necessary.

1. Capitation is neither simply doing what was done in the past in a more complicated way nor a recipe to maintain income and the status quo. It represents a new interdependence between good providers and good payers for mutual benefit. As a result, the practice of medicine should

no longer be a "contest" between payers, providers, and patients for the maximal reimbursement and services, respectively. Instead, capitation should shift and restore the focus of care from the provider's and payer's interests to those of the patient, based on appropriateness. Oversight and rewards must be present to ensure appropriate use and prevent underuse of services (8).

2. The payer or managed care organization (MCO) that is part of this interdependence must be a partner with the physician. There must be mutual trust and a willingness to share data about the demographics of the population at risk, their prior medical activity, as well as past and real time utilization statistics. In the precontract phase, this will help the physician understand the potential impact of capitation on the practice. Subsequently throughout the relationship, this will help the doctor assess the equity of reimbursement for the services rendered. Real-time electronic linkage is crucial, and both parties must have this capability.

   In addition to data sharing, the financial viability of the MCO must be assessed in relation to current and past performance in the marketplace. Obtain a copy of their annual report and read it critically. Don't just look at the pictures! Analyze profit and loss numbers, cash flow, growth, debt, and reserves. Be satisfied that they are economically strong, with the likelihood that they will be in business in 10 years.

   When you are satisfied with economic stability, nonfinancial issues must be explored. A knowledge of the MCO's past track record in dealing with physicians, their driving-force philosophy (dollars or quality), and their ability to provide adjunctive tools for success (electronic linkage, case management, alternative site support) should be consciously assessed and graded. If the organization has not been supportive or responsive in these areas in the past, it is not likely that a long-term capitated arrangement will be philosophically compatible with your practice. Assessing and understanding the quality of the health plan is a most important early step.

   To complete this fundamental database, talk with providers who have dealt with the MCO in the past. Ask whether payments have been prompt and accurate. Have reimbursement changes paralleled changes in premiums and the cost of living? Have they been able to talk with a physician executive about important clinical issues and directions?

3. The physician must be critical and analytical of the practice's ability to function under capitation. Because the promise of capitation is some degree of market share, can the practice handle an influx of new patients with the current personnel and computer systems? Does this "market share" represent new patients or merely a shift of an existing population? Decisions about practice size and additional partners or

support staff are required today in preparation for the "offer" of capitation. Decisions must be based on facts, not last-minute guesses.

Crucial to this process is the assessment of the world around the practice. It does not exist in a vacuum. If you receive some of the market share, will it be at the expense of your colleagues and peers? You may now become their enemy, with resultant social, communal, or even referral isolation.

4. Before concluding any capitated arrangement, the physician must join the ranks of other businessmen and understand what it costs to deliver the product. Before a shoe manufacturer sells a pair of shoes, he knows manufacturing and distribution costs and then prices his product to make a profit. Physicians generally neither know what it costs to see a patient in the office nor understand the economics of additional sessions of office hours, etc. Doctors need to know what it costs them to "make the shoes" before negotiating with anyone.

5. It is impossible to provide a detailed education about contracts in this chapter. Any capitated arrangement should be reviewed by a lawyer before consummation. However, several universal principles should be understood and resolved before the lawyers get involved. They include

Exclusivity—will you be the only physician in the network?

Duration—is this a long-term arrangement so that you can make long-term decisions?

Termination—can you get out if the arrangement is not satisfactory and can you be replaced without cause? Remember that any language that gives you the ability to end the relationship easily will be reciprocal.

Scope of service—what services are included in the capitation rate? What services are your responsibility and which belong to the MCO? A listing of CPT codes clearly defines responsibility.

Withholds—is any money being held from the capitation rate for out-of-area care, "carve-outs," the care provided by other capitated physicians, or any other reason?

Copayments—is the member responsible for any deductible or copayment when care is provided? Can you "balance bill"? In general, the latter is not an option, and a knowledge of the patient's deductible and copayment responsibility is essential to understand the economics of the offered capitation rate.

Membership—in addition to demographics and the plan's ability to provide that information, it must be clear how payment is made when the initial membership is low. A small capitated population is accompanied by a chance for adverse selection. This may result in provision of a disproportionate amount of services for the actual capitation reimbursement. To offset this risk, there are several alternative payment options that might coexist until a critical number of capitated patients is reached. These are discussed in the risk section below.

6. Future success will depend on understanding the concept of risk. How much risk is the practice willing to take and how much risk is the payer willing to give? In general, risk and financial gain are directly proportional. At the lowest level, risk is limited to time and its value compared with full risk for all services and care at all sites. To start, *(a)* define the risk and delineate the scope of services and responsibility for each component and *(b)* develop a mechanism for protection against small membership selection—either fee for service until a critical number is reached or some form of stop-loss protection. The latter, as insurance, is generally less expensive to purchase from an independent insurer than to purchase against your capitation from the MCO.

Formation of Networks

Networks are a fundamental component of managed care. They can be impaneled by the MCO, with defined criteria for inclusion/exclusion, or develop independently (single or multispecialty) to contract with an MCO. This is not a friendly phenomenon for the solo practitioner. I doubt that there is a future for these providers unless they have a unique skill or expertise to fill a void in the existing participating physician network. Even then, the attraction and contracting will be with networks. Thus, the solo physician who cannot provide all-inclusive services and/or has limited geographic coverage ability presents little attraction for MCOs.

Every physician must make a decision regarding practice size and relationships. At its simplest level, a link to a physician hospital organization or an independent practice association may suffice. Depending on your area's practice climate or your specialty, linkage with a single specialty or multispecialty practice may be an alternative. Trading a minimal loss of independence for a guaranteed future access to patients may be reasonable. The decision guidelines regarding practice size, type, and choosing a group are comparable to those about capitation and joining an MCO; they require the same degree of research and vigilance, and like MCOs, ultimately, everyone will not be invited or included, so part of that preparation is also learning to market your practice.

Another form of consolidation and network formation is practice acquisition. The shift from independent practice to a salaried employee status has mixed implications. On one hand, there is a guarantee of security for a predetermined (negotiated) duration, you can just practice medicine and not be an administrator, and the buying organization representing you may be a more powerful and attractive entity to the MCO. The trade-off may be loss of autonomy regarding multiple aspects of your professional life: practice style, work ethic, and colleagues.

Regionalization of "High-Tech" "High-Cost" Services

A reasonable body of literature implies that low-volume providers have different outcomes than high-volume providers (9–11). With everything else being equal, outcomes that are better than expected after severity adjustment provide a major competitive advantage in the marketplace. Develop expertise, gear your practice to focus work in that area, concentrate volume, track your performance, and begin to market yourself. Become known as the subspecialist to whom the specialists refer. To complete the "package" calculate the costs of this service and develop a competitive all-inclusive case rate as part of that marketing approach. If you can objectively show that you provide the best outcomes, efficiently and at a lower price, there is no way that anyone can logically avoid working with you. The experiences at regional "centers of excellence" reflect the ability to decrease cost and increase quality when outcomes and costs are measured (12–14). As classical business principles begin to dominate the marketplace, value (the combination of cost and quality) will dominate.

The Shift of Service Site from Inpatient to Outpatient

Mature managed care markets experience a shift in service site to the outpatient setting. This places an added incentive and emphasis on "office practice" and reduces the focus of the hospital. In turn, this forces three major practice decisions: can you expand your office-based services, should you continue to provide care for your hospitalized patients, and should you develop strategic relationships with hospital-based physicians so that you can remain in the office? Any services that you can develop in your office or through your office that bypass the hospital should be attractive to the MCO. This means developing the capability to provide services traditionally defined in the hospital setting, e.g., intravenous fluid infusion at the primary care level and endoscopy, cardioversion, and minor surgery at the specialty level.

For practices that are hospital based, it is important to spread your risk. All of the current institutions will not be present 10 years from now. With a reduction in the size and number of hospitals, logic dictates that independent practitioners maintain active staff privileges at more than one hospital. Repeat the exercises previously defined for managed care organizations and physician groups and begin now to evaluate the quality of the current hospital leadership, the institution's past and current economic track record, its ability to be flexible and respond to the environment, and your overall perception of its viability.

Use of Nonphysician Caregivers

Many of the services currently delivered by physicians can be performed equally well, with high levels of patient satisfaction, by non-physicians (15, 16). Nurse midwifery is an example. In conjunction with physicians, much of well baby and child pediatrics, primary care, and routine screening in specialty medicine can be performed by advanced practice nurses or physician assistants. With direct supervision and as part of a collaborative system of health care, quality can be maintained, and this should not represent "second-class" medicine (17, 18). In fact, this becomes an effective strategy to maximize access to care, maximize physician effectiveness, and reduce the cost of "routine" care. Examples of the latter include basic screening and health maintenance services, care that meets the inclusion criteria of well-defined clinical pathways, and proactive patient-management programs for multiple diseases. This will involve a new team composed of an office-based facilitator making outbound contact (either by telephone or computer) and a nonphysician clinician alternating individual and group teaching/counseling sessions with visits for disease education and management—linked and probably employed by the practice rather than outsourced to an agency as in today's environment. This team approach can also be applied to help reduce length of stay for hospitalized patients and to improve postdischarge compliance and quality of life (19, 20). In the future there will be an expanded acceptance of this practice mode not only by physicians but by patients and insurers. The economic advantages of adding a nonphysician rather than another physician partner are significant and must be considered as future practice is defined.

Paradigm Shifts

Being proactive in the delivery of care requires a shift in mentality and office capability. Systems and personnel will identify populations at risk. Once identified, a standardized and comprehensive set of guidelines will be applied in management. For example, in addition to patients with overt congestive heart failure, those high-risk diabetics, survivors of myocardial infarction, etc. without clinical manifestations of heart failure will be identified and targeted for proactive disease management. All identified participants will be severity adjusted and placed on protocols that are category specific. Being ready for the future requires this change in doctor focus from watchful waiting to identification, outreach, and preventive intervention. Begin to develop your own pathways or implement existing accepted pathways today. Start on a small scale with a single common disease. Be creative and use a multidimensional approach to deliver care (21). As you become more adept, expand the scope for that disease and add another. Track your results and apply the classical principles of continuous quality improvement (CQI) to do it better over time. The important thing is to begin now and not wait for an imposed mandate forcing implementation under pressure. As you proceed, measure what you have accomplished—not only for CQI, but for marketing and the promotion of your practice.

An Implied Overabundance of Specialists

It is impossible to predict the ultimate direction of specialty care. Most current models interpose the primary care physician as gatekeeper and coordinator of care between the patient and the specialist. There is no reason to believe that this model will be significantly different in the future. Will the only gatekeeper be a primary care physician or will a "generalist specialist" provide the access to subspecialty care? These two scenarios have major implications for the required number of specialists in the future. Many national organizations advocate reduction in the ratio of specialists to the population at risk (22). Projections of 1 per 10,000 to 1 per 40,000 for the number of specialists, depending on the insurance model and the specialty, have been described. Regardless of the model, the primary care physician will maintain control over access to specialty care. Dealing with this complex issue is discussed in the "Specialty Care" section below.

Measurement of Outcomes and Physician Report Cards

Performance reporting is a reality (23, 24) and part of the public domain (25). Acceptance of the concept, understanding what is being measured, and the pitfalls of the measurement process are crucial for the future. Several recent reviews have described the problems associated with measurement and profiling (26, 27). Purchasers of health care, government agencies, hospitals, and MCOs are under either economic, competitive, and/or legislated pressure to compare physicians and the care that they deliver. Measurement can be externally imposed or internally driven. The former is usually based on somewhat limited or incomplete data sets such as claims or encounter data. The latter has the potential to more accurately reflect performance when based on actual chart review and clinical outcomes data. Both require validation; both require strict and universally applied definitions, standardized information gathering, and uniform reporting criteria for acceptance; both require case mixing or severity adjustment; both require the input of multiple objective parties of varied expertise (insurer, clinician, statistician) to define, track, and interpret parameters.

Patient satisfaction has been an early and almost universal measurement tool (28). Although questioned by some as a reliable mirror of physician performance, patient surveys have been shown to correlate with other parameters of performance and outcome (29). In any event, this information is vigorously sought by purchasers of health care and is a major focus of all health plans' measurement activity. Recently, peer ratings of physician performance have been described (30).

Other measurements such as the Health Plan Employer Data Information Sets (HEDIS) are based on common measurable variables. HEDIS 2.5 includes more than 60 parameters of performance (31). Although initially applied to health plans, many of these indicators are now being used by those organizations to rate individual physician performance and to guide reimbursement. Data are collected and reported according to strict and well-defined criteria to ensure uniformity and comparison between health plans. Similar definition and uniformity will ultimately be extended to many more specialty- and subspecialty-focused parameters for future network decision making. That this exists even in an embryonic form may be a revelation to many physicians. The first step in preparation is acknowledging that the future practice of medicine will depend on these outcomes. The second step is an understanding of the parameters, adjusting practice patterns to meet and exceed current published benchmarks, tracking individual and practice results, and remaining flexible for floating-endpoint targets and new parameters.

Individual accountability is with us to stay. As stated in other sections of this chapter, decisions about purchasing health care insurance, physician participation in plans and networks, and the ability to perform procedures and testing will be based on comparative outcomes data. Therefore, begin to work with your colleagues, hospital, and/or dominant MCO to develop tools to track and measure your practice's performance, as a marketing tool and as a defense when you do not agree with the data that are presented about you by any third party.

COMMON ISSUES

In preparation for the future practice of medicine, there are several common questions for each practitioner. The best advice is to learn to ask the right questions and to recognize change. Each answer and solution will be individualized, resulting from the interplay of the trends and realities previously discussed. For now, only the questions should be posed, the right answers will vary depending on when and where the questions are asked. Begin the planning process by asking yourself the questions listed in Table 16.2.

Although there are many common issues and adaptations, there are several areas where primary care physicians differ from specialists and academic medical center (AMC) physicians differ from non-AMC-based physicians.

Primary Care

The role of the primary care physician as gatekeeper and coordinator of care continues to be an essential and fixed element of managed care (32). The need for these physicians will probably increase as more of the population comes under a managed care umbrella, including those millions not presently insured. The threat to future survival and economic up-

Table 16.2
Practice Assessment Questions

Practice type
• Do you want to practice alone or in a group?
• If in a group, should it be primary care only, single specialty, or multispecialty?
• Do you want to employ nonphysician caregivers as part of the practice?
• Do you want to remain independent or be acquired by an outside group?
• If acquired, do you work for a hospital, an insurance company, or another middleman?
• If acquired, who will be the policymaker for the way that you will practice regarding working conditions and clinical decision making and what ancillary support relations exist?
• How much and how many managed care arrangements do you want?
• How much risk can you take now and will you be willing to take in the future--assuming that you understand the risks and benefits of taking risk.
• Do you want to practice in an academic medical center? If yes, how are you going to divide your time between patient care, education, and research?

Individual clinical issues
• What are your strengths and weaknesses?
• How can you minimize your weaknesses and capitalize on your strengths?
• What new skills are you likely to need to be successful in the next 5, 10 years?
• What are you doing today that is passé, based on anecdotal experience and countercurrent to the present and future direction of medicine?

Practice mechanics
• Where can you cut administrative costs and manage the practice more efficiently?
• What should you be measuring?
• How can you more effectively market your practice to patients and insurers?
• What data systems and personnel are needed to achieve these goals?

heaval is therefore less for this group than for specialists. Success will be directly proportional to understanding and adapting to payment models that emphasize appropriate behavior: understand the model and then tailor your practice to take advantage of its incentives. If there are multiple MCOs with different reimbursement models, look for common performance measures and act on them, with an emphasis on the principle payer's model. In the future, it may become impossible to successfully contract with all carriers, especially if they value different skills and services, impose different clinical pathways, laboratories, and ancillary service providers. Ultimately, you might have to make a choice and limit your participation to fewer payers, but for the present, keep all options open and wait to see how and who defines the marketplace.

Regardless of the number or type of surviving MCOs, preventive skills will be more highly valued in the future, whether as a criterion for participation or as part of a compensation model. It no longer is sufficient to wait for people to only "show up" when they have a problem. Outreach and prevention must be emphasized to be successful. Prepare now and develop the mechanisms to identify, provide, recall, and track a full range of age-specific preventive services. This change in practice focus may require a reallocation of resources or even additional physician and/or physician-extender personnel along with sophisticated data tracking and recall systems. If your practice is not computerized or electronically linked to payers, correcting this deficiency should become your number one priority.

Equally important is the ability to communicate with your patients prior to and between visits to your office. This has at least two practical implications. As you teach your patients your practice style, they will become "better patients," and you can be more efficient in delivering care. This may even limit emergency room visits and improve your managed care utilization. This can be accomplished with general and specific practice newsletters and brochures to introduce your patients to the nuances of your practice.

Effective communication also teaches a new disease-management paradigm to make your patients more knowledgeable partners in care delivery. The model already exists for patients with diabetes who measure their sugars regularly and adjust their insulin accordingly, with improved control of their blood sugars and an enhanced quality of life (33). They understand their disease and participate actively in its management. This concept should be extended beyond diabetes to similarly involve your patients in the management of a wide spectrum of chronic illness.

With an emphasis on prevention and being proactive, hospital admissions and stays are reduced. This makes you more attractive to an MCO. In addition, most managed care contracts include hospital care in the primary care scope of services. In the future, it is likely that this care will be an optional carve-out. With more resources devoted to outpatient medicine, will you maintain the skills or inclination to provide hospital care to your patients or will these services be subcapitated, subcontracted, or referred to a hospital-based doctor? As discussed above, it is likely that in the future, distinction will be made between office- and hospital-based physicians. The latter are generally more cost-effective and -efficient, with outcomes that are equal to or better than the "mixed" mode that currently dominates for the care of hospitalized patients.

This efficiency is an incentive to create a group practice. Other advantages of a group over solo practice are listed in Table 16.3, and the incremental advantages of a multispecialty group are listed in Table 16.4. Both models increase access to care, improve efficiency, increase choice, and provide incremental attraction to MCOs.

Specialty Care

The organization of specialists into large single and multispecialty groups is growing. Compared with the primary care community, there is much more uncertainty among specialists regarding their viability. As managed care replaces traditional fee-for-service reimbursement with capitation, income is threatened because smaller networks are created to provide care. Everyone wants to participate, and it is clear that everyone

Table 16.3
Advantages of a Group Practice

Coverage
Peer review
Internal consultation
Enhanced patient choice and access
Continuity and increased ability to provide hospital care
Larger patient base with more likelihood of collecting statistically significant outcome data
Economy of administration

Table 16.4
Advantages of Multispecialty Models

Aligned goals between primary care and specialists
Ease of access to specialty care
Clear continuity of care
Internal education
Curbside consultation capabilities
Enhanced member satisfaction with "one-stop shopping"
Ease of communication

will not participate in the future. A basic requirement for inclusion is the capability to provide full service in a specialty or across specialties to a wide geographic area.

How can you be attractive to a "group" in this redefined environment? For long-term success, it has to be more than just willingness to accept a reduced fee. As the shift to the classic principles of economics emerges, price and quality need to be aligned. Success will depend on objectively demonstrating that better skills, clinical judgment, and patient outcomes can be delivered in a cost-competitive manner. Specialists who do not exceed community standards and performance targets will neither be valued nor participate in networks. This is especially true as networks begin to take financial risk. As long as there is no risk, organizers are happy and willing to take "everybody." When there is risk, only the proven better performers remain attractive. It is our job to be sure that "better" is well defined on the basis of objective measures of quality (access, appropriateness, outcomes, and patient satisfaction) rather than just lower cost.

How then will the marketplace distinguish among specialists, beyond cost? Ultimately, this will depend on development of broad-based performance measurement and "report cards." Today, the first cut in differentiating specialists is board certification. Purchasers and certification groups (National Committee for Quality Assurance) request and make decisions based on the percentages of specialists that are board certified. Therefore, MCOs seek this information and make network inclusion/exclusion decisions on the basis of this single criterion—it is objective and makes a network inclusion distinction. Further subdivision of the network requires additional objective performance measurement with well-defined and validated criteria.

Therefore, to remain in a pool for network consideration, board certification (and subspecialty certification if it exists) is crucial. It is the single most important deficiency to correct as soon as possible. On a parallel track, begin to gather data and measure your performance.

If the first requirement for future success is to be included in a network, the second requirement is to have access to patients. As stated above, for most models, this is through the primary care physician. For integrated multispecialty groups, capturing lives is not a problem. Your partners, the primary care physicians, have created a base for you. For single specialty groups or individuals, the key is also the primary physician and his or her decision to include you in patient care. To market to this force, you need to distinguish yourself in the network from your colleagues. You have to show the primary care physician that you do a better job and provide better service than the alternative choices. Assuming that your competition is indistinguishable on the basis of report cards and performance measurement, what can you do? Communication is the key, and you should begin today to do a better job. The following four maneuvers will help to cement a lasting relationship with primary care physicians.

1. Let all of your referring primary care physicians know how important they are to you. Meet them and find out how you can serve them better. Learn what they need and expect. Face to face, discuss how you both can work together more effectively. The better you meet their needs, the more solid the relationship.
2. Provide information about patient contact in a "super timely" manner. Fax results and reports the same day as consultation, and make it a habit to communicate on the telephone regularly.
3. Become an educator. Teach your specialty to the primary care physician. This has a major effect on your credibility, especially while there is still a fee-for-service component. Tell them that they can do more at their level, and give them parameters to ensure appropriate referral. In the long run, they will be better physicians, and as capitation grows, this will limit inappropriate "dumping." Also be a patient educator and provide the environment for patients to participate in interactive decision making (34). This has been shown to reduce costs and improve patient satisfaction and all providers' status with MCOs.
4. Let the primary care physician know your strengths and weaknesses. Let them know what you do best, and do not be afraid to urge them to use another specialist who may have more expertise in a subspecialized area of your specialty. For example, as an orthopaedic surgeon, your expertise may be hip or knee replacement, with only average results for the infrequent shoulder replacement. Somebody else clearly has more expertise and better outcomes with this surgery. Let your primary care physician referrer know that for that particular patient, the "other guy" does a better job and should perform the surgery rather than you.

From an economic standpoint, you can be more successful and enhance your attraction to the MCO and primary care physician by developing the capability to perform diagnostic testing and minor procedures in an alternative outpatient setting. Quality and safety must be equal to or exceed the results of the hospital. A partial list of outpatient alternative-setting procedures is listed in Table 16.5.

Another controversial issue is retraining. If indeed, there are too many specialists, then retraining for primary care may be necessary. MCOs clearly define the requirements for primary care. Not all specialists have the requisite skills and qualifications to make an automatic transition from specialist to primary care physician, e.g., not all general surgeons will be acceptable to a managed care organization to provide primary care. A

Table 16.5
Alternative Setting

SPECIALTY	PROCEDURE(S)
Gastroenterology	Endoscopy, liver biopsy
Cardiology	Catheterization, EPS, cardioversion
Pulmonary	Bronchoscopy
Nephrology	Renal biopsy
Heme-Onc	Chemotherapy
Orthopaedic surgery	Arthroscopy
Urology	Endoscopy, vasectomy
General surgery	Minor surgery, lumpectomy
Ob-gyn	Laparoscopic surgery
Ophthalmology	Minor surgery including cataracts
Otolaryngology	Endoscopy and endoscopic surgery

standard definition of "retraining" does not currently exist. This issue will be hotly debated over the next few years. If you perceive that you will ultimately need to practice in a primary care role, I suggest that you contact the dominant MCO in the area and find out what they require for you to assume that role. Be proactive and do not wait for the "ax" to fall before preparing.

Academic Medical Center

A comprehensive discussion of AMCs has been recently published (35, 36). Major concerns stem from a decrease in funding for education and research compounded by the fear that the AMC can not be competitive in a marketplace potentially driven by cost alone. For future success, physicians based in an AMC must also become accountable and competitive. No longer will reputation alone drive referrals and ensure access to patients. Based on case mix adjustment, the data must prove better outcomes and expertise and justify any incremental cost compared with community-delivered services. The major adjustments for future positioning combine accepting a job description with emphasis on patient care, honing clinical skills that may have been dormant for some time, marrying an academic focus with the practical realities of cost-effective medicine, and learning to interact and communicate with referring physicians.

Physicians in AMCs are further disadvantaged because of the inherent higher costs associated with these institutions because of case mixing, education, research, and underlying inefficiency. Competing against talented community hospital–based physicians will be difficult—it is more expensive to perform a simple cholecystectomy in the AMC than in "Community General." In spite of equal physician reimbursement, the outcome will be the same, patient satisfaction may actually be better in the community (closer to home, parking, no residents to bother them, etc.), and the overall cost is clearly more in the AMC. Physicians and the AMC must follow the same exercise as the office-based physician, i.e., understand what it costs to deliver a service, reduce unnecessary excess, and increase efficiency without sacrificing quality. Concurrently, define and market the abundant subspecialty expertise that uniquely exists in the AMC.

FINAL SUGGESTIONS

It is impossible to ask all of the questions and provide the checklist that will ensure success for the future. Rapid changes in the environment may yield a world that is unimaginable, even in the short time from writing to publication of this chapter. However, here are my "best-guess" preparation suggestions with universal applicability.

- Do not focus on the past and "its glory." The good old days are gone.
- Become computer literate. The future will revolve around electronic information dispersion.
- Understand what you do best and begin to do it better.
- Remain medically current and creative and provide the best care possible.
- Be an educator and teach your patients to be more healthy—turn your waiting room into an educational room.
- Regularly survey your patients about their satisfaction and to find out what you don't know about your practice; follow their suggestions for improvement.
- Establish standards of care and introduce clinical pathways.
- Begin today to track common procedures and diseases related to your practice, prospectively with an understanding of severity adjustment.
- Only track parameters that you control.
- Monitor admissions and review what could have been avoided both for the individual patient and for changing practice patterns in general. Make changes to avoid those admissions in the future.
- Choose one target diagnosis for length-of-stay reduction and develop the tools and skills to make it happen.
- Partner with a nurse group and provide proactive management of chronic disease.
- Market yourself and don't be afraid to disassociate yourself from the poor performers who will drag you down in the long run.
- Choose a managed care partner wisely. Join and work with them as a participant. Learn about managed care as an insider and from the inside.
- Cut waste and administrative costs.

- Do not be passive, remain flexible, and continually reevaluate the market place and your position in it.

CONCLUSION

Returning to Dickens, "it was the age of wisdom, it was the age of foolishness." Overall, I am optimistic for the future. However, we are still living with an element of foolishness: long-term planning for physicians today is valid for no more than 18 months at most. The world is rapidly changing. To provide the metamorphosis to an age of wisdom, follow the "triple open policy": keep your eyes open to a changing environment; keep your mind open to rational change and be flexible; keep your options open and do not commit yourself to any process, group, or contract until you are sure that it is right for you.

We can have more control over our destiny and patient care than ever before. Medicine wedded to appropriateness and accountability with a new proactive focus will give us the ability to alter the natural history of disease in a manner never before imagined, to create the "best of times in a age of wisdom."

REFERENCES

1. Dickens CA. A tale of two cities, p.1.
2. Schreiber G, Poullier J-P, Greenwald L. US health expenditure performance: an international comparison and data update. Health Care Financ Rev 1992;13:1–15.
3. Inglehart JK. The American health care system-managed care. N Engl J Med 1992;327: 742–747.
4. Murray D. The four market stages, and where you fit it. Med Econ 1995;72(5):44–57.
5. Teisberg EO, Porter Me, Brown GB. Making competition in health care work. Harvard Bus Rev 1994;4:131–141.
6. Wachtel TJ, Stein MD. Fee for time system: a conceptual framework for an incentive neutral method of physician payment. JAMA 1993;270:1226–1229.
7. Diamond GA, Denton TA, Matloff JM. Fee for benefit: a strategy to improve the quality of health care and control costs through reimbursement incentives. Am J Cardiol 1993; 22:343–352.
8. Hillman AL. Health maintenance organizations. Financial incentives, and physicians' judgments. Ann Intern Med 1990;112:891–893.
9. ACC/AHA Task Force Report. Guidelines and indications for coronary artery bypass graft surgery; a report of the American College of Cardiology/American Heart Association Task Force on assessment of diagnostic and therapeutic cardiovascular procedures (Subcommittee on Coronary Artery Bypass surgery). J Am Coll Cardiol 1989;17:543–589.
10. Laffel GL, Barnett AI, Finkelstein S, Kaye MP. The relation between experience and outcome in heart transplantation. N Engl J Med 1992;327:1220–1225.
11. Ritchie JL, Phillips KA, Luft H. Coronary angioplasty in California in 1989 [abstract]. Circulation 1992;86(suppl):I-1011.
12. Boyle MH, Torrence GW, Sinclair JC, Horwood SP. Economic evaluation of neonatal intensive care of very low birth weight infants. N Engl J Med 1983;308:1330–1337.
13. Showstack JA, Rosenfeld KE, Garnick DW, Luft HS, et al. Association of volume with outcome of coronary artery bypass graft surgery: scheduled vs. nonscheduled operations. JAMA 1987;39:148–151.

14. Gordon TA, Burleyson GP, Tielsch JM, Cameron JL. The effects of regionalization on cost and outcome for one general high risk surgical procedure. Ann Surg 1995;221:43–49.
15. Sox HC Jr. Quality of patient care by nurse practitioners and physician's assistants: a ten year perspective. Ann Intern Med 1979;91:459–468.
16. Maule WF. Screening for colorectal cancer by nurse endoscopists. N Engl J Med 1994;330: 183–187.
17. Ginsburg JA, Sox H Jr, Ginsberg JA, Denman Scott H, et al. Physician assistants and nurse practitioners. Ann Intern Med 1994;121:714–716.
18. Yawn BP, Jacott WE, Yawn RA. Minnesota Care (Health Right): myths and miracles. JAMA 1993;269:511–515.
19. Moher D, Weinberg A, Hanlon R, Runnalls K. Effects of a medical team coordinator on length of hospital stay. Can Med Assoc J 1992;146:511–515.
20. Levetan CS, Salas JR, Wilets IF, Zumoff B. Impact of endocrine and diabetes team consultation on hospital length of stay for patients with diabetes. Am J Med 1995;99:22–28.
21. Litzelman DK, Dittus RS, Miller ME, Tierney WM. Requiring physicians to respond to computerized reminders improves their compliance with preventive care protocols. J Gen Intern Med 1993;8:311–317.
22. Schroeder SA, Sandy LG. Specialty distribution of U.S. physicians—the invisible driver of health care costs [editorial]. N Engl J Med 1993;328:961–963.
23. Hannan EL, Kilburn H Jr, O'Donnell MA, Lukacik G, Shields EP. Adult open heart surgery in New York state: an analysis of risk factors and hospital mortality rates. JAMA 1990;264:2768–2774.
24. Welch HG, Miller ME, Welch WP. Physician profiling: an analysis of inpatient practice patterns in Florida and Oregon. N Engl J Med 1994;330:607–611.
25. Zinman D. Heart surgeons rated. State reveals patient mortality records. Newsday 1991;Dec 18:34.
26. Topol EJ, Califf RM. Scorecard cardiovascular medicine: its impact and future directions. Ann Intern Med 1994;120:65–69.
27. Epstein A. Performance reports on quality—prototypes, problems, and prospects. N Engl J Med 1995;333:57–61.
28. Kaplan SH, Ware JE. The patient's role in health care quality assessment. In: Nash DB, Goldfield N, eds. Providing quality care. Ann Arbor, MI: American College of Physicians, 1989:11–25.
29. Schlackman N. Integrating quality assessment and physician incentive payment. QRB 1989;15:234–237.
30. Ramsey PG, Wenrich MD, Carline JD, Inui TS, Larson EB, LoGerfo JP. Use of peer ratings to evaluate physician performance. JAMA 1993;269:1655–1660.
31. Report Card Pilot Project. Key findings and lessons learned: 21 plans' performance profiles. Washington, DC: National Committee for Quality Assurance, 1995.
32. Franks P, Clancy CM, Nutting PA. Gatekeeping revisited—protecting patients from over treatment. N Engl J Med 1992;327:424–427.
33. Greenfield S, Kaplan S, Ware JE, et al. Patient participation in medical care: effects on blood sugar control and quality of life in diabetes. J Gen Intern Med 1988;3:448–457.
34. Kasper JF, Mulley AG, Wennberg JE, Developing shared decision making programs to improve quality of health care. QRB 1992;18:183–190.
35. Inglehart JK. Rapid changes for academic medical centers. Part 1. N Engl J Med 1994;331:1391–1395.
36. Inglehart JK. Rapid changes for academic medical centers. Part 2. N Engl J Med 1994;332:407–411.

INDEX

Page numbers followed by "t" refer to tables.